THE CANCER SURVIVAL GUIDE

Practical Help, Spiritual Hope

KAY MARSHALL STROM

Beacon Hill Press of Kansas City
Kansas City, Missouri

Copyright 2002
by Beacon Hill Press of Kansas City

ISBN 083-411-9749

Printed in the
United States of America

Cover Design: Kevin Williamson

Library of Congress Cataloging-in-Publication Data

Strom, Kay Marshall, 1943-
    The cancer survival guide : practical help, spiritual hope / Kay Marshall Strom.
        p. cm.
Includes bibliographical references.
    ISBN 0-8341-1974-9 (pbk.)
    1. Cancer—Patients—Religious life. 2. Cancer—Religious aspects—Christianity.
I. Title.
    BV4910.33 .S77 2002
    248.8'6196994—dc21

                                                                2002003221

10 9 8 7 6 5 4 3 2

CONTENTS

INTRODUCTION

Cancer. It's the terrifying disease we all pray we'll never get. We think we know a fair bit about it because there's information everywhere, but the facts are hopelessly tangled up with myths and out-of-date information. What we do know is that many people seem to get cancer and then they die.

First the bad news: Current statistics warn us that one out of every three people in the United States will develop the disease. It's the No. 2 killer after heart disease, and it's rapidly threatening to take over the No. 1 spot. No amount of money or success can prevent or stop it. The fact that you've just had a baby or a grandchild, fallen in love, gotten that big promotion you've been working toward, finally built your dream house, or figured out how you can retire early—it doesn't matter one bit. Nothing does.

And the good news? Cancer, once considered so hopeless a diagnosis that some people wouldn't even utter the word out loud, is becoming less formidable. Many new and exciting therapies are being tested throughout the world, especially in the United States. Besides numerous new drugs—more powerful and effective yet with fewer and lighter side effects—we're seeing such scientific breakthroughs as stem cell transplants, gene splicing, enzyme inhibitors that choke off the blood supply to tumors, genetic and molecular technologies that trigger cancer cells to die, and a number of applications of new studies on DNA. Many types of cancer that were routinely considered a death sentence less than 20 years ago are now curable. And many more advances are in the works. We have every reason to believe that the progress against cancer will be even more dramatic in the years to come.

It gives all of us reason to hope.

Mine is a family touched by cancer. This week my mother celebrated her fifth anniversary of being cancer-free. Her mother and grandmother were not so fortunate. My husband, Dan, and I, relative newlyweds, both lost our first spouses to death, his to cancer and mine to a rare degenerative genetic condition by the daunting name of neuroacanthocytosis. We are well acquainted with illness and loss.

But that's not what this book is about. Nor is it about all the exciting possibilities in cancer detection and treatment. That information, which changes almost daily, can be readily found in a number of other books and periodicals. Rather, this book is about God and how He deals with His children in the most difficult of circumstances. It's about how He alone sees the end from the beginning and how He works every detail of our lives together for our good and His glory. For people who are dealing with cancer, the coping process is far more than merely physical. It is, first and foremost, spiritual.

Author and theologian C. S. Lewis in his book *A Grief Observed* wrote, "You never know how much you really believe anything until its truth or falsehood becomes a matter of life and death to you."[1] He had the right to speak; he watched helplessly as bone cancer consumed the body of his beloved wife, Joy.

God wants us to freely choose to believe and love Him, even when that choice involves suffering and pain and questions we can't answer. He wants us to cling to Him simply because we're committed to Him rather than to whatever else might provide us with better feelings and comfort and immediate reward. He wants us to hold tight even when it seems we have every reason to turn away from Him and cry, "My Father, why have You forsaken me?"

Good can come from the ugliest and most devastating of circumstances. Mind you, I'm not saying that the circumstance itself is good—not the cancer or the neuroacanthocytosis or any other thing that causes suffering. What *is* good are the changes that take place in us while we walk through the darkness, the changes that give unmistakable evidence of the presence of God. Who but God himself could enable us to endure a fear and agony too deep for words and come through it with rejoicing on our lips and hope in our hearts?

God provides the grace we need in the hour we need it, not one day earlier and not one day too late.

In Heb. 4:16 we read, "Let us therefore draw near with confidence to the throne of grace, that we may receive mercy and may find grace to help in the time of need" (NASB).

Come along as we begin that journey of confidence to the throne of grace.

1
THERE MUST BE SOME MISTAKE!

It was just two days before Christmas, and Myra Mahoney was running around in circles. There were cookies to bake, Christmas dinner to plan for all the relatives who would be coming to town, shopping to do, gifts to wrap. And there were church choir and school pageant rehearsals, and—oh, yes—her yearly physical exam. Myra always scheduled her physical in December. That way she wouldn't forget it, and it would be done before the end-of-the-year insurance deadline.

Myra's physical included a routine trip to her gynecologist. As it turned out, that trip was anything but routine. During the examination the doctor discovered a lump in the wall of her colon. "I knew immediately something was very wrong," she says. "There's no way a person can have a lump there without it being bad. Some places, yes, but not there."

The doctor knew it too. Suddenly he was scurrying here and there, making notes, checking this, and rechecking that. "I could tell he was trying not to scare me, even as he insisted I go *immediately* to see a surgeon—like *now!* He made a telephone call right then and there, and 45 minutes later I was in the surgeon's office."

Scared and confused, Myra telephoned her husband, Tim. She needed him with her in case she found out something terrible. The surgeon, a specialist in colon surgery, examined her and confirmed what the other doctor had found. Yes, he said, there definitely was a lump. Myra

stared into his face, trying desperately to read the significance behind his words. But his face remained calm. It
seemed to say, *It's not that bad. It's going to be OK.*

But it wasn't OK. Myra, a 45-year-old mother of two active boys. Myra, who felt perfectly fine and was far too
busy to be sick. Myra, who trusted God, prayed, studied
her Bible, and did her best to live for the Lord.

Myra had cancer.

Shock. Disbelief. Terror. Then the sudden realization
that nothing would be the same again. Not ever!

Christmas preparations screeched to a halt as a parade
of doctors and tests and lab reports began. Confused and
uncertain, she and Tim decided not to tell anyone except
their kids about the diagnosis.

The surgeon informed her that they had a picture of the
tumor. Now they had to figure out how to get a biopsy of it.
But it could wait until after Christmas, he assured her. Go
home, he said. Have a happy holiday. Season's greetings.

Myra couldn't think straight. Her mind played games
on her and sent her imagination reeling. It was just too
much to take in. Too much.

"Don't worry," Tim assured Myra. "It won't be cancer.
It's going to turn out to be nothing at all. You'll see."

Myra looked her husband straight in the face and said,
"You're wrong, Tim. It can't be 'nothing at all.' I fully expect it to be cancer."

Two days after Christmas, Myra had the biopsy. Only
she and Mark, her 15-year-old son, were home when the
telephone rang the next afternoon. Even before she picked
up the receiver she knew what she would hear.

"Myra," the receptionist said, "the doctor is in the operating room, and he asked me to see if you're home, because he wants to call you."

It wasn't going to be good news. Myra sat and waited
by the telephone for the doctor's call.

It came within minutes. "I just got the results from the
lab," he said. "You have squamous-cell carcinoma, possi-

bly metastatic. We have identified the exact position." With his matter-of-fact voice and his technical language, the doctor sounded eerily like an emotionally removed scientist. "You are going to have to go over to the cancer center and get a little bit of chemotherapy and a bit of radiation."

"What?" Myra exclaimed in exasperation. "I don't understand what you're saying here. I know carcinoma is cancer, but what exactly are you telling me?"

What he was telling her was that the type of cancer the biopsy had revealed—squamous-cell carcinoma—is a type found on the skin and sometimes in a few other places in the body, but never in the colon. That meant the cancer had likely spread from somewhere else in her body. If it had indeed started somewhere else, then her colon was only one of the places she had it.

"That was the worst part of the whole ordeal," Myra said. "My son stood right there, seeing and hearing everything." Hardly able to hold herself together, she first called Tim at work. She knew he was going to fall completely apart when he heard the news.

Tim's response was "I'm coming home right this minute."

Then Myra picked up 9-year-old Kevin from school so that the whole family could try to take this in together.

EVERYONE REACTS

Everyone reacts to life-changing news in his or her own way. Some remain distant and removed, as though the matter is not really of that much concern. Others refuse to accept the situation, insisting there's some mistake. Some break down in inconsolable emotion, others determine to remain stoic, while still others are too numb to react at all. Some people lash out at God in anger, demanding an answer or at least an explanation. Others fall on their knees before Him begging for mercy and a miracle. A few just give up in resignation.

Tim reacted with a flood of tears. "This can't be happening!" he insisted. "It simply can't be! I can't raise these boys by myself!"

Mark showed his pain and shock at the news, but Kevin did not. Myra assumed he was too young to really grasp the significance of what was happening. But that wasn't so. A counselor from his school called and told Myra that Kevin was talking about it at school nonstop, telling everyone, "My mom has cancer." She suggested it might be wise to get him some counseling.

Myra had her own way of reacting: head-on and matter-of-factly. "We have lots of people counseling us already," she told the school counselor. "I know this is serious, but I truly don't think I'm going to die. Thank you for your concern. If we need more help, we'll call you." Any help Kevin was to receive, Myra determined, would come from people who shared their Christian point-of-view.

Tim's father reacted to the news in a get-the-job-done businessman sort of way. "I'm sending you two first-class airline tickets," he told Myra and Tim. "I want you to go anywhere in the world you need to go to have this taken care of. Don't worry about the cost—just get it fixed. Everything's going to be OK."

Myra was especially surprised at how her sister, to whom she was especially close, took the news. "It's going to be OK, Myra—it really is," she said calmly and confidently. What Myra didn't know until much later was that as soon as she got off the phone, her sister broke down and sobbed uncontrollably.

It's important to understand and accept that people will react differently. No one should be criticized or judged for not reacting the way another person does or in a way someone else expects that person to. Until we're in that position, none of us really knows how we would respond.

Take Justin's family, for instance. Justin, a successful type-A businessman, had been diagnosed with a brain tumor that was very likely malignant. The day before his surgery, his family held an all-day get-together at his home and a special dinner with all his favorites. Although he appreciated having his family around him, the day was awkward and exhausting. His son, who came from graduate school in another state to be there, seemed irritable and angry the entire day. Justin's wife, Nancy, acted as though nothing was wrong and insisted on laughing, telling silly stories, and chattering on about unimportant things. His daughter kept her distance, burying herself in work in the kitchen.

"I couldn't talk to any of them," Justin said sadly. "I longed to tell them how scared I was and how much I love them all and what I wanted them to do if I didn't make it, but no one wanted to hear it. So I, too, tried to pretend nothing was wrong and that my son was just in a bad mood and my daughter was in a funk. But when I went to bed that night, I cried myself to sleep."

FROM FEAR . . .

Wise King Solomon would have this reassurance to offer Justin: "When you lie down, you will not be afraid; when you lie down, your sleep will be sweet" (Prov. 3:24).

Most of us would respond, "You aren't facing reality, Solomon. You obviously have no idea of what fear is!"

Actually, he did. So did the apostle Paul when he penned these words to the suffering Christians in Rome: "You did not receive a spirit that makes you a slave again to fear, but you received the Spirit of sonship. And by him we cry, 'Abba, Father'" (Rom. 8:15).

When we face something so fraught with ominous mystery as cancer, we *do* feel afraid, even we who love and trust the Lord. It's our human nature. To deny it forces us to suffer in silence. How much better it is to face the fear, to express it openly, and then turn it over to God. Ps. 46:1—which promises: "God is our refuge and strength, an ever-present help in trouble"—is not a mere platitude. It is the truth.

How do we know? Because we have God's promise of everlasting protection. Just look at these verses of holy Scripture: "He [God] will cover you with his feathers, and under his wings you will find refuge; his faithfulness will be your shield and rampart" (Ps. 91:4). "I am the LORD, your God, who takes hold of your right hand and says to you, Do not fear" (Isa. 41:13).

. . . TO PEACE

You say it's not natural to find peace in the midst of a diagnosis of cancer? No, it isn't. That's why we must tap into the supernatural peace of God through Jesus Christ. It was Jesus himself who said, "Do not be afraid, little flock, for your Father has been pleased to give you the kingdom" (Luke 12:32).

In the face of such news, there's no peace unless it comes from the Lord.

"Everyone acted like I was going to die," Myra says. "Some people even told me so. Others just told me awful stories with sad endings, but I knew exactly what they meant."

It seems to be human nature to recall the most dramatic and tragic of stories. And it's true that where cancer is concerned, our minds tend to reel with unhappy endings. The perception of the finality of a cancer diagnosis is hard to shake, although we're beginning to gain a more realistic understanding of the possibilities. In a couple of months my daughter and I will be taking part in a three-day walk to help raise breast cancer awareness. The wonderful thing about this event is that while some people, such as Lisa and I, are walking in the name of a survivor (we're walking on behalf of my mother), the majority of the participants are themselves breast cancer survivors. There's every reason to be hopeful.

Still, you're entering the world of the unknown. How far has your cancer advanced? What will the chemotherapy do to the cancer and to your body as a whole? How about those other terrifying sounding treatments? You may not know, but you know the One who has the answers.

"If I were to go home to be with God, I knew full well that I would be going to a far better place," Myra said with conviction. "But I didn't want to die. There were so many things I still wanted to do and accomplish. I desperately wanted to continue in my relationship with my husband. And I hated the thought of my children being hurt and having to grow up without a mother. I really, really wanted to live! And so it brought me great peace to know that God was with me and understood my fears and my desire to survive."

Peace in the diagnosis of cancer. Peace in the face of treatments prescribed and debated. Peace despite all the fearsome stories and dire warnings. Everything familiar and secure is gone. The unthinkable reality sets in—and yet there's peace.

We're taken by surprise, but God never is.

You're helpless, but you have God's unlimited strength to fall back on. There are decisions that need to be made, treatments to be decided upon, a whole new medical language to be learned. Yet through it all, underneath you, supporting and sustaining you, are God's everlasting arms.

God Knows You

With that pronouncement of "You have cancer" and the flurry of tests and procedures and doctors that follow, you may begin to feel transformed from an individual with a name and a family and an entire life into just a cancer patient—or even worse, just "colon cancer." It isn't true. Don't believe it for a single minute. You are the special, individual person God created you to be. You can say with the psalmist David, "I praise you [God] because I am fearfully and wonderfully made; your works are wonderful, I know that full well" (Ps. 139:14).

You say you're worried and concerned about the days ahead?

Of course you are. But God will not forsake you. He hears your pain and knows your fear, and He waits to comfort you through His Word.

2

No More Business as Usual

You always assumed life would go on as usual. Like all of us, you lived expecting that the important circumstances of your world would pretty much stay the same. Now this has happened, and your cancer diagnosis is all consuming. You find it difficult to concentrate on anything except the disease and what it will mean to you and your family.

"I admit it—I've always been a control freak," Justin said.

It was important to me to be in control of my life and everything that touched it. Then one day I woke up with one eyelid sagging so badly I had trouble making my way down the stairs to the kitchen. I tried to ask my wife what she thought was wrong, but my speech was so slurred she could hardly understand me. She rushed me to the emergency room, and before the day was over I had been told I had a brain tumor that was probably malignant, and I was scheduled for surgery the following morning. Just like that. No one asked me—they told me. One day I was the most important man in the office, and the next I couldn't even open my eye or speak intelligibly. One day I refused to ever take a day off work because I was certain they couldn't get by without me, and the next I didn't give the company a second thought. One day I was in control, and the next I was totally at the mercy of those around me.

No more business as usual.

IF ONLY . . .

After the day-long flurry of tests and scans and doctors and nurses, Justin's wife was ordered home to get some rest, and he was alone in his private room. Despite the sedatives, he lay in bed thinking. Recalling that long and agonizing night, he says, "I'm a full-blown type-A personality, a businessman who worked long and hard to get where I was. There in that bed, so helpless and vulnerable, I was plagued with questions: Was the cancer caused by all my cell phone use? Was it my long hours of work? Was it because I never felt I could afford the time to take a vacation? What was it I had done wrong to bring on brain cancer?"

Justin is not alone in his questions. Many people look at their cancer and ask, "Why?" Very often, that very understandable question is quickly followed by "If only . . ."

If only I had taken better care of myself.

If only I had gotten my yearly checkups.

If only I had eaten a healthier diet.

If only I hadn't smoked for so many years.

If only I had lost weight.

If only I hadn't spent so much time in the sun.

If only I had taken vitamins.

If only I had walked a mile each day.

If only . . .

McCall's magazine printed an article in March 2001 titled "Hit the Health Jackpot." The first two sentences state, "The evidence is in: Whether you get cancer is largely within your control. Even if your genes predispose you to the disease, how you live your life has more influence on your odds of cancer striking than your DNA."[1]

Whoa! Pile on the guilt!

The "if only" guilt is especially strong in people who suffer from a somewhat preventable disease such as lung cancer. We all know about the warnings on cigarette packages. In many states we see clever and poignant television spots that warn of the dangers of smoking. Parents who smoke are nagged by their children to quit. We've heard the statistics that tell us that nearly 90 percent of lung cancer cases are smoking related. So when a person is diagnosed with lung cancer—well, here's what 69-year-old Theo has to say: "I was a smoker most of my life. I'm ashamed to say I was just too weak to quit, even though I knew I should. I totally blame myself for my cancer. I smoked even though I knew better."

Yes, Theo should have quit smoking. But if we haven't walked in his shoes, we can't know how difficult that may have been for him. He says he was *totally* at fault for his disease. Totally? Really? What about the tobacco companies who seem to target young people? Like the 80 percent of smokers, Theo started using cigarettes when he was a teenager. What about the romanticized view of smoking with which we're still presented in the movies and by advertisers? What about his parents, who modeled smoking throughout his childhood and his teen years? What about his wife, who was an even heavier smoker?

Guilt and self-blame do nothing to help us fight cancer. Whether or not our "if onlys" have some validity or none at all, holding onto endless guilt keeps us from moving on. It prevents us from throwing ourselves into the things that now need to be done.

Whatever the level of validity, regrets and self-blaming cannot change what is. If you allow yourself to wallow in guilt and remorse, you'll surely sink into despair. You have cancer. Accept that reality. Then, with God's help, get ready for the fight of your life.

For good or for ill, a diagnosis of cancer is likely to set off a period of intense soul-searching. Suddenly, forced to come face-to-face with our own mortality, we pause to take stock of our lives. When you look closely at yourself, are you pleased with what you see? Or does your soul-searching fill you with regrets?

Self-examination is demanding, but it's also rewarding. Yes, it pulls us up short in the face of our failures, and that's definitely painful. But it also awakens us to all kinds of new and exciting possibilities. Yes, it convicts us of our guilt. But it also leads us to grace.

So What Now?

No more business as usual. Instead, we have many new matters of business to take up, many new questions to ask and considerations to ponder. Think of this as *the new approach.*

Will you have surgery? Over half of all cancer cures result from surgery alone. How about radiation? In many people, it can shrink a tumor to where it can be dealt with more effectively. Chemotherapy? Yes, you've heard horror stories about it, but its benefits are unmistakable and can, in fact, be quite remarkable. Chemotherapy is the foundation of treatment for many, many cancer patients.

All these treatments, especially chemotherapy, are very different from what they were as recently as five years ago. The new drugs are significantly more effective and in many cases much less toxic. And oncologists are able to administer them in a way that minimizes side effects while still obtaining the greatest benefit. Side effects are fewer and less intense than in the past. Radiation is more limited in scope and surgery less invasive.

A major part of your new approach will be to learn all you can about your particular cancer, to listen carefully to the advice of your doctors, to weigh the various possibilities with your family, and—most important—to lay it all out before God. Trust Him to guide you, and give Him complete control.

Don't worry that you'll be struggling alone through your treatment. You'll be amazed at the number of loving, caring people, organizations, and groups that are ready and willing to help.

"When the doctor scheduled me for surgery so quickly, I was terrified," Justin recalled. "I didn't want to do something so drastic without first doing a little research, and certainly not before talking it over with my family. Yet I could just see that tumor growing by the second!"

Justin, stunned and confused, asked the doctor straight out if the surgery had to be done so quickly. Immediately the doctor slowed down the schedule and assured him that a few days would make no difference at all.

If at all possible, slow down your decision-making. Sure, you feel a sense of urgency to decide what you're going to have done and who's going to be involved in doing it. You may also be eager to look into the pros and cons of herbal supplements and vitamins, alternative treatments, and your diet in general. Determine which decisions have to be made immediately and which ones can wait awhile. Act immediately and decisively where you need to; then slow down and gather information and support where you can afford to move more slowly.

Whatever the urgency, don't allow yourself to be frightened or pressured into making decisions about your treatment until you're sure you have a clear understanding of your choices. Ask about and explore the options. Take time to pray and wait upon the Lord. Search the Scriptures. In many cases, if you back off a bit, you'll not only be able to make better decisions but also have much greater peace of mind.

A major step toward achieving a positive revised approach is to get over your desire to keep your diagnosis a secret. Once you conquer this, you'll be surprised at how much support and positive feedback you will get. Ken, a survivor of prostate cancer, is an energetic supporter of moving past the secrecy. "Once I was open about my cancer, I started getting a steady stream of E-mails. And as I progressed through the various stages, I sent updates to my family, friends, and colleagues. It was so great to know I wasn't alone. The feedback was critical to helping me maintain a positive attitude, and I'm convinced that maintaining a positive attitude is vitally important when you're facing surgery."

Also, by being open about where he was, Ken discovered people he knew who had faced the same situation. By sharing their stories, they offered a special kind of support and provided him with information that helped ease his fears and offered him concrete guidance.

Today Ken says exactly the same thing he so often said in his E-mail messages: "I'm truly blessed to have such loving, supportive friends. And should I need any additional support in the future, I know without a doubt they're still there."

Jeremy Geffen, M.D., in his book *The Journey Through Cancer* wrote, "I've found that the true miracles of cancer rarely take the form of drugs, potions, or herbs. More often than not, the true miracles take place in the minds, hearts, and spirits of patients and their families."[2]

I'm sure that to some degree that's true of all cancer patients, but for Christians it's absolutely central. It's the miracles that heal, and it's the miracles that bring us in line with the mind of Christ.

Consider Jesus' example. When facing the Cross, He prayed, "Father, if you are willing, take this cup from me; yet not my will, but yours be done" (Luke 22:42). Christ was facing something He could not change and still remain true to the redemptive purpose of God the Father. There was no other way. He simply had to endure the horror of the Cross.

It's when we have no choice but to endure that we need to cling tightly to Heb. 4:16 and to hold it close to our hearts: "Let us then approach the throne of grace with confidence, so that we may receive mercy and find grace to help us in our time of need."

It's this mercy and grace that will help us endure the roller-coaster emotions that are sure to hit.

3
ROLLER-COASTER EMOTIONS

"Surprise! We're having a 30th high school reunion cel- ebration!" announced a couple of women who had been friends of Tim and Myra's since junior high school.

"What?" Myra asked. "Two years early?"

"We're not going to wait," they said. "You know . . . just in case you don't make it."

The celebration lasted all weekend. On their last night in the hotel, the group of friends sat together in the lobby, laughing and talking into the wee hours of the morning. It was just like old times. Laughing so hard she had to gasp for breath, Myra clutched at the neck of her purple velvet high-neck top. "I've got to stop laughing, guys! My chemo catheter is hurting!"

Everyone froze in midlaugh. No, perhaps it *wasn't* just like old times.

One week later Myra celebrated her birthday. Not your usual celebration, however. Chemotherapy started that day, along with radiation treatments. Tears ran down ev- eryone's faces as the shadow of fear of the unknown hov- ered over the day.

Celebrations and preparations. Life and its threat of an untimely end. Fear and hope and then more fear. Anger and acceptance. After receiving a diagnosis of cancer, the ups and downs of conflicting emotions threaten to over- whelm even the strongest among us. Those roller-coaster emotions sneak in from all directions, unexpectedly turn- ing smiles to tears. They jerk you first to the right and then to the left. They surge, they wane, they explode, they fade. They leave you confused and exhausted.

Myra didn't even try for a long-term viewpoint. "If I could just make it from one step to the next without dying, that's all I focused on," she said. "Just one step. Then one more. Next week, next month, next year . . . I would deal with that when I got there."

Good advice. But it doesn't happen easily, not when you're looking death in the face.

A Cycle of Emotions

It's no secret that our emotions can have a profound effect on our bodies, just as the condition of our bodies can affect our emotions. No wonder a diagnosis of cancer brings on an emotional roller-coaster ride! There are sure to be times when you want to scream, times you'll cry, and—believe it or not—times you'll sing out praises to God.

Although no one progresses through this emotional abyss in an orderly fashion, there are certain emotions you can expect.

Shock. *Cancer? It can't be! It just isn't possible!* Myra's 80-year-old friend next door was waiting on pins and needles to hear the diagnosis, so Myra ran over to break the news to her. When she got back home, Tim was already there. She had intended to be there for him when he came in the door. He was in such distress he couldn't even talk.

"This can't be happening!" he sobbed. "You do *not* have cancer!" Before Myra could respond, Tim exclaimed, "Don't worry, Myra—don't worry. It's going to be OK. There's a mistake. It's not going to be anything."

"You're wrong, Tim," she said. "There is no mistake—it *is* cancer."

Shock is an understandable first emotion, both for you and for your family. It's a hard one to escape. Sometimes that shock is actually heightened by the doctor.

"Even after the diagnosis of brain cancer, I was doing pretty well," Justin said. "Then I sat in the doctor's office, and he said, 'It will be a miracle if you're alive in a month.' Talk about shock!"

Fear. When she began to comprehend the seriousness of her cancer, Myra asked the doctor straight out, "Am I going to die?" He immediately answered, "No." Then he quickly stepped back and qualified his answer. The fact was, he didn't know. No one did.

How far has the cancer advanced? Can it be cured, or will it kill you? How will your body react to the treatment? No one knows the answers to those questions. The unknown: that's the first part, and for some people it's the most terrifying part.

But there are other fears as well:

- The cancer may change my life forever.
- It may be terribly painful.
- The treatments might cause me awful suffering.
- The disease might have a really bad effect on my family.
- I may not be able to cope with the disease.
- My joy of living may be gone forever.

"I hadn't just lost control of my body," Justin said. "I had lost control of my life."

Fear of losses. The fear of having your life yanked out from under you. The fear of suddenly feeling powerless and vulnerable.

Yet in the midst of your fear, a promise from God: "Do not fear, for I am with you; do not be dismayed, for I am your God. I will strengthen you and help you; I will uphold you with my righteous right hand" (Isa. 41:10).

Anger. "Angry?" Theo said. "You bet I was!" He was angry at everyone—his doctors, the nurses, his wife, his family, his friends. And he was furious at God.

"All day I bellowed and bullied. But at night, when no one could hear or see, I cried in misery."

Actually, anger is one of the most common reactions to

serious illness. And very often, ill persons take the anger out on those closest to them.

Grief. Before Myra started her treatments, she and Tim went away for an overnight stay together. Tim told her, "I want you to know, if you die I'm not going to get remarried until the kids are grown up. I don't want to have to blend a family." Only a couple weeks had passed since the cancer was diagnosed, and they were already beyond crying. But they were not beyond sadness.

"Sadness was a major emotion for me," Myra said. "I felt very, very sad a good deal of the time."

You, too? Then the following invitation is especially for you. It's from Jesus Christ himself: "Come to me, all you who are weary and burdened, and I will give you rest" (Matt. 11:28).

Guilt. It must be my fault. I must have done something to cause this.

Again, this is a classic emotion. You ate too much junk food and too little broccoli. You drank too much coffee. You didn't exercise enough, or correctly, or in the right way. You used water right out of the tap. You didn't wash your hands often enough.

Some people wrestle in silence with their guilt. Tim came right out and asked the doctor, "How could this have happened to my wife?" The doctor looked him straight in the eye and said, "It's not because of anything she did or you did."

Sometimes the answer isn't quite so easy. Let's look again at Theo:

"My family tried everything to get me to stop smoking," he said, shaking his head at the memory. "When my daughter was seven years old, she made me a Father's Day card that said, *Plese, plese, plese don't smok, Daddy. I don't want you to die!* I kissed her and assured her that Daddy wasn't going to die. Then I lit up another cigarette. Today I see the recrimination in my daughter's eyes when she looks at me and at the pain I've put her mother through.

I'm sad, and I'm suffering, but most of all I'm feeling guilty and angry at myself."

Shock. Fear. Anger. Grief. Guilt. All very real emotions. All legitimate. All understandable. Don't let anyone tell you how or how not to feel. Denying your emotions, holding your feelings in check because you want to be strong, or to prove your trust in God, or because you think you have no right to express them can be extremely detrimental to your recovery. Feelings are not right or wrong. It's what you do with them that's good or bad.

So what's a good way to handle your feelings? Acknowledge them. Express them. Refrain from criticizing yourself for them. Look at the way God regards your emotions: "Record my lament; list my tears on your scroll—are they not in your record?" (Ps. 56:8). The King James Version puts it this way: "Put thou my tears into thy bottle."

The Lord God, ruler of the universe, tenderly collects the tears you shed. He saves them all and records each of them in His eternal record! That, dear friend, is how important your emotions are.

So what's a bad way to handle your emotions? Wallowing in them. Allowing them to take over your life. Permitting them to plunge you into bitterness and despair.

Linda watched helplessly as her husband, Keith, sank further and further into this way of showing his emotions. Angry since he was first told about his liver cancer, he soon expressed that anger as blame, which he directed against his wife. She was the source of so much stress in his life, he claimed. And she "never cooked worth a hoot. It's a wonder we aren't all sick!" Keith and Linda have three children, two of whom are teenagers. They also received a double helping of Keith's wrath: "Noisy, selfish, self-absorbed—just like all kids today."

Keith's bitterness also turned to cynicism toward God.

"I wish I could share Scripture verses with Keith," Linda said sadly. "I wish we could talk together about the comfort packed in those pages. Maybe in time."

One verse Linda is looking forward to sharing with Keith is Ps. 22:24—

> He has not despised or disdained
> the suffering of the afflicted one;
> he has not hidden his face from him
> but has listened to his cry for help.

Despair. There's one more emotion we need to talk about—despair. Please understand—despair has nothing to do with your faith or lack of it. You have cancer. It's a big deal. It's forcing you to look at a whole lot of difficult things at a most inconvenient time. You can be quite mature in your faith and well-grounded in Scripture and still experience despair. No matter who you are, when you come face-to-face with death, it takes time to grasp the stark reality of your own mortality.

You have only to look to the Book of Psalms to see that David, the man after God's own heart, was no stranger to despair. The same is true of the other psalmists of the Bible. In Ps. 42:5-7, the writer clearly states that his soul is downcast. The thing is, he doesn't stop there. No, even in that condition he clings to his faith and hope in the Lord. He remembers how God has faithfully cared for him in the past, and this assures him that God is trustworthy now as well. He didn't have to see it or feel it to know it was true.

Neither do you. Like men and women before you, you can find comfort and courage by remembering God's faithfulness in the past—to you, your ancestors, the saints throughout the ages, the patriarchs. Then you, too, can shout verse 11 in triumph:

> Why are you downcast, O my soul?
> Why so disturbed within me?
> Put your hope in God,
> for I will yet praise him,
> my Savior and my God *(Ps. 42:11).*

How utterly incredible! And you can put your hope right here even when your feelings betray you.

The journey from despair to faith may be short or it

may be long. At times it will be difficult. But you don't have to make it alone. Ask the Lord God to help you along. And when your resources are gone, ask Him to carry you through the darkness into the light.

Marlene has been living with cancer for 22 years. She was only 36 years old when she was first diagnosed with breast cancer. "In the first five years, I suffered so badly from despair that the doctor had to give me medication for it. The thing was, I wanted answers, and I wanted assurances. When I couldn't get them, I plunged into a deep depression. It took me years to come to where I could take one day at a time. Who would have thought 22 years ago that I would live to see my children grow up and marry and raise children of their own? I'm 58 years old, and I fully intend to live to see my great-grandchildren!"

The difference between despair and hope has nothing to do with your cancer. It has everything to do with the decisions you make about what you'll do from this day forth. You can't change the situation, but you can allow the situation to change you—for the better.

Acceptance

There's a huge difference between resignation and acceptance. Resignation is surrender to blind fate. Acceptance is surrender to a loving God. Resignation lies down and gives up. Acceptance rises up to meet the purpose for which God created the person. Resignation says, "I can't. It's all over." Acceptance says, "I can't, but God can!"

We fight hard to do things our way. Acceptance is giving up our way and trusting God to guide us. It's saying with the psalmist: "As for God, his way is perfect; the word of the LORD is flawless. He is a shield for all who take refuge in him" (18:30).

And acceptance propels us forward to our everlasting hope in the Lord.

HOPE

Whatever part of your body is affected by cancer—brain, breast, prostate, lung, stomach, liver, ovaries, testicles, colon, skin, bones, throat, blood—even if your entire body is riddled with cancer—no one has a right to say, "Yeah, you're going to die." Only God decides who lives and who dies. No human being, not even the most renowned cancer specialist in the entire world, can know that. Doctors have been proven wrong far too many times.

We're not talking about people who staunchly refuse to accept the diagnosis of cancer. Denial isn't hope—it's foolishness. But remember Justin, who was given weeks to live? Well, the doctors were wrong. That was three years ago, and he's in remission and is doing great. He's back at work, and while he's still an A-type personality, he no longer is so driven or, in his own words, "such a control freak."

"I refused to be a statistic," Justin says with deep passion. "I'm an individual like no other individual who has ever lived or who ever will live. And I'm proud to say that, despite the dire predictions, I'm a cancer survivor!"

Here's something that may help to get your emotions in control: *Cancer is not a death sentence.* No matter how crummy you feel, no matter how dire your prognosis, *it's always too soon to give up!* There's no cancer from which nobody has recovered. Recovery is *always* a possibility. There's every reason to hope. You can be realistic, you can be accepting—yet never, ever be afraid to hope.

Here is a mantra for you to type out and post on your bathroom mirror, by your coffee pot, in your work station at the office, on your refrigerator door, tucked into your wallet, on the dashboard of your car, or anywhere else you won't be able to miss it:

I have hope!
If anyone can make it, with God's help, I can!

After acceptance comes hope. And after hope comes peace.

PEACE

Peace? When you're suffering from cancer? It doesn't make sense!

Right you are. It doesn't make sense because peace doesn't come from logic. It comes from the Holy Spirit. (See Gal. 5:22.)

Only God can give you peace in the midst of turmoil. As the apostle Paul wrote in Phil. 4:7, "The peace of God, which transcends all comprehension, will guard your hearts and your minds in Christ Jesus."

Jesus himself had some comforting words on this subject: "I have told you these things, so that in me you may have peace. In this world you will have trouble. But take heart! I have overcome the world" (John 16:33).

THANK YOU, GOD, FOR THE ROLLER-COASTER RIDE

If you allow it to, this back-and-forth, up-and-down roller-coaster ride of emotions can give you three pretty great gifts:

- It can open the door to hard questions and force you to listen to the answers.
- It can reveal the spiritual direction in which you are heading.
- It can drive you to your knees before the Lord.

We're mortal beings. Unless the Lord returns first, every one of us is going to die. All in all, it isn't such a bad thing to have our phony illusions of mortality profoundly shaken. Sure, it's terrifying. But it can also be an opportunity to have a transforming experience in ourselves, in our world, and before our God. It gives us a push toward learning and growing in ways we never imagined possible. It may make an enormous difference in how you and I live each day from now on.

Your cancer can well be the gateway to a very different life!

4

THE GOOD, THE BAD, AND THE SCARY

Insist that God heal you!
Repent of your sins and you'll get well!
God won't give you more than you can bear.
You think you have it bad? Listen to what I had to go through!
I have a friend who knows a guy whose sister has a treatment that can cure you.
If you just have enough faith . . .

Suddenly advice pours in from all sides. Everyone—at work, at home, in the neighborhood, in the pews at church —seems to feel a duty to offer his or her two cents' worth.

And then there are the books by cancer survivors. Some did one thing, and some did another, but the message always seems to be the same: *Do it my way and live! Refuse to give up and survive! Whether you live or die is your responsibility. It's all in your hands.*

Hardest of all are the ones who purport to speak for God. Some follow in the footsteps of Job's friends and insist, *Confess your sins, turn from your wrong ways, and you'll be healed.* Others declare, *God chose you, just as He chose Job, to be an example. Others are watching you, and their faith depends on how you handle this.*

And you're left to cry, "What am I supposed to do? What's the lesson I'm to learn in all of this? How much more faith can I muster when I'm being battered on all sides?"

ENCOURAGING WORDS

From those who should have been the most encouraging, Myra received a surprising amount of discouragement. Still in shock, she presented her situation to her church and asked the congregation for prayer. After the service, a woman she hardly knew approached her and announced, "All doctors know how to do is cut you and burn you. They killed my daughter, and they're going to kill you!"

Shocked and confused, Myra asked her pastor, "What am I going to do? How am I ever going to get through this?"

Although the pastor was upbeat and encouraging, Myra hardly heard anything he said to her. She couldn't get the faces of the people in the congregation out of her mind. "Everyone had tears in their eyes," she says, "and I knew why. They were all convinced I was going to die."

That's not how it should be. The psalmist wrote, "You hear, O LORD, the desire of the afflicted; you encourage them, and you listen to their cry" (10:17).

The apostle Paul took the idea of encouragement a step further when he wrote to the Christians at Rome, "May the God who gives endurance and encouragement give you a spirit of unity among yourselves as you follow Christ Jesus, so that with one heart and mouth you may glorify the God and Father of our Lord Jesus Christ" (15:5-6).

That's how God's children are to respond to those in need of encouragement.

And for Myra, there were those who did.

A cancer survivor was in the congregation that day, a man by the name of Charlie. Yes, his experience was different from Myra's. For one thing, he had a totally different type of cancer—prostate. But even in cases in which the type of cancer is the same, everything surrounding the approach and treatment might be completely different. So it makes little sense for one cancer sufferer to share advice on treatments with another. But that wasn't Charlie's approach. Instead of advising, he provided the words of encouragement Myra so desperately needed.

"My doctors told me I didn't have a chance," Charlie told her. "They said the cancer had progressed so far that there was nothing they could do."

Charlie told Myra that when he heard that diagnosis, he fell apart. He actually crumbled up and sobbed. But after allowing himself some grieving time, he picked himself up and got to work. After a great deal of research, he found the absolute best place in the country for the treatment of his type of cancer. Since the doctors hadn't been able to give him hope, he promptly volunteered for any experimental therapy in progress. He was accepted for a trial type of radiation. It just so happened that the specialty equipment needed for the treatment was located 100 miles from his home. So every single morning for six weeks, Charlie took a train to the treatment center, went through the radiation, and then rode the train back home.

"The thing is, with God's help I made it," he told Myra. "And you'll make it too. Praise the Lord!"

Encouragement.

A spirit of unity.

Giving glory to God the Father and to our Lord Jesus Christ.

Myra had cried out to her pastor, "What am I going to do?" and up stepped Charlie with wonderful words of encouragement that could have come right out of the Book of Romans.

Myra's experience demonstrates a wonderful assurance each one of us can claim: "Before they call I will answer; while they are still speaking I will hear" (Isa. 65:24).

Encouragement comes in many shapes and through many people.

Again and again Myra heard the dire warning "If you have chemotherapy, it will kill you." She never knew how to answer. She did have Charlie's example to hold on to, but with so many people telling her otherwise—well, it was just too confusing, not to mention emotionally upsetting.

"I didn't know how to respond to them," Myra says. "I didn't want to be impolite. And I didn't want to cut them off; after all, they may have had some really important information for me. But . . ."

But all that negative input was quickly wearing her down. Tim could see what was happening to her, and he stepped in with a different kind of encouragement: active intervention. Early one morning, long before the sun was up, Tim was at his desk hard at work. First he read every one of Myra's books on cancer. Then he set about putting together a business plan for fighting her disease. When Myra awoke, he handed her an official-looking folder of papers, all neatly printed out and clipped together.

"Here's the plan," he said. "Now when someone comes up to you and says, 'You should eat brown rice,' or 'Drink lots of grape juice,' all you have to do is refer to the plan. If it's not here, you're not eating brown rice or drinking lots of grape juice."

Myra read over what he had written, and she liked it. It was agreed: anything that wasn't on the plan would not be considered.

"That really helped," Myra says. "Even if I never looked at that plan again, it gave me something to say to everyone who wanted to give me advice. Now I had an answer."

You cannot afford to be an emotional wreck right now. It takes too much out of you to be pushed this way and that by everyone's opinion and advice and warnings. The best protection is to have an answer ready. When people come up with unsolicited advice, tell them you already have a course of treatment charted for yourself, and you really don't want to discuss it. If a person won't respect your wishes, say goodbye and leave. Or hang up the telephone. Or go into your bedroom and close the door. Or don't take that person's calls.

I know, I know—you don't want to be rude. But look at it as giving yourself the protection you need.

Even with the plan, one woman just wouldn't take Myra's "no" for an answer. After pushing her alternative plan again and again, she walked up to Myra and handed her a 15-page fax listing all the dangers of chemotherapy. Each point had terrifying anecdotal "evidence" to support it. Finally Myra could take no more. "I got really mad and ripped that thing up. I just said, 'Hey, I'm not doing this! I don't want to talk about it any more, and I don't want to hear any more about it!' And I walked out on her."

Did that woman ever talk to Myra again? I don't know. Does it matter? Absolutely not.

Tim's wisdom in designing the cancer treatment business plan became abundantly clear when Myra encountered Teresa, a woman her age who was dying of the very same type of cancer Myra had. The doctors had assured Teresa, "We can cure you of this; here's what you need to do." But Teresa had heard too many horror stories and had listened to too much unsolicited advice. So she turned away from the doctor's prescribed treatment and instead tried to do all the things everyone else told her to. She ate vegetables and drank juice and had coffee colonics and took herbs and relaxed and visualized the good cells wiping out the bad cells. When it became obvious that this approach wasn't working, she went back to the cancer center. But by then her cancer was too advanced. She died soon afterward.

People may mean well, but meaning well is not the same as speaking and doing well. If someone is harming your ability to fight the cancer in your body, you need to stay away from that person. For Justin, that person was Stan, an acquaintance from a men's retreat he had attended several times. Stan fancied himself gifted by God to identify and cast out demons. And when he appeared on Justin's doorstep unexpected and unannounced, that is exactly what he was determined to do. Trying to be polite and patient, Justin allowed Stan to come in, and for a few minutes they visited and recalled their experiences at the retreat. Then Stan looked Justin in the eye and said, "The problem is that you have a demon, Justin."

Ignoring Justin's weak protests, Stan proceeded to "pray the demons out" of Justin, then out of the house. Afterward, he triumphantly pronounced Justin healed. "Your cancer has begun to shrink, and as long as you have faith, it will continue to get smaller until it is completely gone," he announced.

As best he could with his slurred speech, Justin explained that he was going in for surgery the next day.

"Oh, no!" Stan exclaimed. "You can't do that! It would mean you don't have faith. You must cancel your surgery and pray!"

Justin's wife, Nancy, who had been doing her best to sit patiently and listen, jumped up and exclaimed, "Absolutely not! Even if Justin wanted to cancel the surgery I wouldn't let him! That surgery can save his life!"

Calmly, Stan looked Nancy in the face. "By not believing, you're killing your husband," he said. "Everyone in the family must believe, or the healing will not take place. Justin must cancel that surgery, and you must support his decision."

Shaking with frustration and rage, Nancy ordered Stan out of the house. Yet that pronouncement hung on. What if he were right? It was very unlikely, but what if . . . ?

After much prayer, Justin and Nancy called their pastor. He sat with them and began by pointing out 1 Cor. 14:33— "God is not the author of confusion, but of peace" (KJV).

Then he read, "Where envying and strife is, there is confusion and every evil work. But the wisdom that is from above is first pure, then peaceable, gentle, and easy to be entreated, full of mercy and good fruits, without partiality, and without hypocrisy. And the fruit of righteousness is sown in peace of them that make peace" (James 3:16-18, KJV).

"Does Stan's wisdom meet this criteria?" the pastor asked.

"No!" said Nancy. "It's anything but peaceable, gentle, and merciful!"

"That's why we have the scriptures," the pastor responded. "They're a guide to help us find our way. Look at Isa. 50:7—'The Lord GOD will help me; therefore shall I not be confounded; therefore have I set my face like a flint, and I know that I shall not be ashamed.'"

Your new business is not to increase your confusion by listening to everyone. It is to rest on God, and in so doing to increase your peace.

PRACTICING MEDICINE WITHOUT A LICENSE

On June 14, 2001, the *Wall Street Journal* printed an article with the headline "Regulators Crack Down on Web's New Miracle Cure: Colloidal Silver." Staff reporter Jill Carroll wrote, "In this age of miracle medicines, here's one that sounds like a real doozy. It's a substance that can cure acne, herpes, cancer, leprosy and the bubonic plague— "more than 650 different disease-causing viruses," its promoters say."[1]

So what is this miracle medical breakthrough? As it turns out, it's actually a centuries-old substance called colloidal silver, and according to the article, federal regulators warn that it's a total scam. Commonly sold in small bottles for as much as $20 per ounce, it's available on an alarmingly large number of web sites.

You'll probably hear about it, as well as a whole slew of other therapies purported to cure cancer. Friends, coworkers, family members—everyone seems to want you to try—and to buy—a whole array of alternative therapies, many of which flourish in places like Mexico and the Bahamas, just out of reach of government regulatory agencies. More than a few are set up for the specific purpose of preying on the desperation of the suffering and hopeless.

Theo was contacted by a classmate he had not seen since high school. "I don't know how Jim heard about me, but he called to tell me that he, too, had lung cancer and that the Laetrile clinic in Mexico was the only reason he was still alive. I was desperate, so I went down there. When I got home two months later, I found out that Jim had died."

Keith was shocked when, at the age of 42, he was diagnosed with liver cancer. The doctors told him straight out that his chances of survival were slim.

When Keith's sister and her husband arrived at his door armed with a video of "someone just like you" who was still alive 10 years later, Keith was eager to hear all about it. That "someone" turned out to be a half dozen personal testimonies attesting to the life-saving properties of Laetrile, coffee enemas, herbal drinks, and other alternative treatments. "Why do so few of us survive cancer?" one woman earnestly asked the camera as she rocked her baby in her arms. "Because too many have too much to gain by keeping us sick!" Then it launched into a warning about a huge conspiracy involving the American Medical Association, pharmaceutical companies, and various cancer institutes. According to the video, they knew all about cures for cancer, but with so much of their money at stake, they weren't about to make that knowledge available to the public.

Keith's wife, Linda, had already walked out of the video show in disgust by the time the earnest woman with the baby came back on to say, "But you're one of the lucky ones. You have someone who cares enough to tell you the truth."

Keith watched until the end, and then he watched it again.

David Sneed, a doctor I once worked with in Austin, Texas, told me, "People need to be very careful about taking anecdotal evidence as proof. Remember: only the living speak." For every person who "visualizes" his or her way to healing or experiences a "miraculous recovery" from herbs, there are thousands more who unsuccessfully tried the same therapies. The difference is that those other people are not around to tell you about their experiences. In his book *The Hidden Agenda,* Dr. Sneed includes the following red flags to watch out for when confronted with an alternative therapy:

1. It takes an unscientific approach.
2. It attempts to make you alone, or "the power within you," responsible for your health.
3. Other authorities aren't familiar with the therapy.
4. It claims that the therapy is a cure-all.
5. It makes claims of extraordinary cure rates.
6. It warns of a "medical conspiracy."
7. The practitioner's explanations don't make sense.
8. Primary proof is from testimonials.
9. It makes claims that reduce the practitioners' accountability.
10. It uses Christian language or endorsements to guarantee legitimacy.[2]

PEOPLE WHO HURT, PEOPLE WHO HELP

"Well," a woman in Myra's Bible study said to her, "you know, God won't give you more than you can bear."

"What?" Myra retorted. "That's not scriptural!"

"Oh, yes it is!" the woman insisted.

Two others chimed in their agreement. Instead of arguing, Myra suggested the women bring the scripture reference to share with her the following week.

They didn't, because they couldn't find it. That's because it isn't there. The oft misquoted verse is actually 1 Cor. 10:13, which reads, "No temptation has seized you except what is common to man. And God is faithful; he will not let you be tempted beyond what you can bear. But when you are tempted, he will also provide a way out so that you can stand up under it."

The fact of the matter is, God absolutely *does* allow you more than you can bear. If He didn't, why would you need

Him? But here, dear friend, is the key: Whenever there's more than you can bear, the Lord God is ready and able to bear *you!*

People don't intend to hurt you. They just speak carelessly. Many don't know what to say. Some are very uncomfortable. They see your pain and feel inadequate to help. They're frightened; if this is happening to you, it could just as easily happen to them too! Some people are well intentioned but misguided. And there always seems to be a few who are so downright thoughtless it's hard to believe.

But then there are the others, the healing people who seem to have just the right words of care and understanding to lift you up and point you toward God.

Whatever their reasons and whatever their intentions, some people are toxic and hurtful while others are healing and comforting.

Toxic People

Toxic people can come from anywhere. They include the woman at church who told Myra, "All doctors know how to do is cut you and burn you. They killed my daughter, and they're going to kill you."

Theo came in contact with more than his share of them. "Everyone thought they were doctors," he said. "They all had an opinion on what I should do. One guy told me, 'You know radiation will just cause the cancer to spread to your brain, don't you?' When I told him I wasn't going to have radiation, just chemo, he said, 'Oh. Too bad. That'll kill you.'"

You would think fellow cancer sufferers would be safe; they would know where you're coming from. Not necessarily. In his book *Hope When It Hurts*, Larry Burkett tells of a young man who managed to get in to see him, approached his bedside, and said, "Larry, I'm a renal cell carcinoma patient also, and you might as well face it: You're going to die. I'm going to die, and you are, too, because there just isn't any cure for this type of cancer."[3]

Even a doctor can be a toxic person. When my mother-in-law was in her late 60s, her doctor told her that the lump she found in her breast was cancer and that her entire breast would have to be removed. When she asked if it was possible to do less drastic surgery, he responded, "What difference does it make? You're an old woman." When we insisted that she get a second opinion, it was discovered that the lump was nothing more than a deep bruise!

What to do about negative people? Let them know that you won't tolerate the negativity. If they can't or won't understand that, get them out of your life. Don't hang around with negative people.

Healing People

You'll also be blessed with people who are ready with beautiful words of encouragement. They're the ones who look you right in the face and greet you with a smile but are really phony, insisting you look great when it's obvious you don't.

Charlie was a healing person. The day Myra told the congregation about her disease, he came up specifically to encourage her to actively search her options. He gave her names and addresses of places to go to seek out the latest research in her type of cancer. He told her his cancer had been considered untreatable but that through research he had found an experimental program, had been accepted, and that the results had been astonishing. "You'll make it!" he told her that day, and in the days to come he was to say it again and again and again.

Justin had a friend who created a web site for him where his wife could post regular updates on his progress so his friends and coworkers could keep current without having to intrude upon the distracted family.

When Emily worried that her children were growing up around her while she was too sick to enjoy them, a friend of her mother, a professional photographer, offered to take a family portrait before she started her treatments.

One young man who works with my husband Dan was diagnosed with a rare form of lymphoma that has a bleak prognosis. His distraught wife sent E-mails to everyone in his address book and asked for prayer for him and their family. Dan passed the request for prayer along to everyone on his E-mail prayer list, which included believers around the world. The young man was moved to tears by this message he received in reply:

Dear Brother,

I am Marcio, a Brazilian Christian who works among unreached fishermen along the Brazilian coastline. My good friend Dan Kline asked me to pray for you. I will be praying not only because he asked me to, but because I am 100-percent sure God wants me to, and to pray for you, my brother, will be a pleasure and a privilege.

You know Brazilians. I want to send you my love, concern, a warm hug, and to remind you that God is always much more interested in what He is doing *in* us than *to* us.

I know the next days will be hard sometimes, but keep on praising God even if you don't understand what is going on. Ephesians 1:5-6 says that we were born to praise His glory, and we don't want to disobey Him, do we?

Feeling with you, weeping a little, and trusting a lot, I remain,

Your Brother Marcio

Embrace those healing people in your life. Hold them fast, and don't let go. It matters not whether they're next door or on the other side of the world.

Oh, and one more thing. Many people talked about the encouragement they received from reading the inspirational stories of other cancer survivors. One suggestion is *Chicken Soup for the Surviving Soul: 101 Healing Stories of Courage and Inspiration.*[4] This book tells the inspiring stories of many others who understand your journey.

HUMAN LOGIC VERSUS GOD'S WAYS

Emily was only 32 and the mother of three young girls when she was diagnosed with breast cancer. "You need to praise God for this," an older woman in the church informed her. "You need to come to the place where you can say, 'God, I *love* You for making me suffer like this. It is Your will. You know the best for me. And I just praise You for loving me enough to allow me to experience this. In all things, including this, I give thanks.'" Emily looked from the woman to her own young girls, and she broke down in tears. "That isn't praising," the woman chided.

Keep reminding yourself that you need not accept all the unsolicited advice from the well-wishers who pass it out so freely. They have never walked in your shoes, and there's no reason to think they have the "right" answers. Who's to say what the right answers are? Everyone suffers differently. Everyone feels pain differently. Everyone expresses emotions differently. Everyone processes differently. Myra did not work through the process the same way Emily did. Theo did not work through it the way Keith did. And you, too, will find your own way.

But don't depend on faulty human logic to show you the way. Rather, take the advice of the writer of the Book of Hebrews: "Let us then approach the throne of grace with confidence, so that we may receive mercy and find grace to help us in our time of need" (4:16).

Want a great promise to cling to, one that's good and true and eternally faithful? Then look at Rom. 5:1-5. Your pain will produce good in your life. It slows you down and forces you to turn to God. It produces character that will keep you from being the ugly, toxic person in another's life. And that's not all: that character produces hope that will never let you down!

5

MAKE YOUR BATTLE PLAN

"Your entire colon needs to be removed," Myra's first doctor informed her. "Yes, the surgery will be rough, and yes, it will leave you with some life-long challenges. But it's your best chance of survival."

Doctor number two didn't agree. He insisted that only the affected area needed to be removed. Problem was, that meant removing a radius of at least one inch around the tumor, and in Myra's case the tumor was less than three-quarters of an inch away from the sphincter. So she would still have to have a permanent colostomy (a surgically built opening in her abdomen through which body wastes are excreted into an attached bag). At 45 years of age and with Myra's bursting-with-energy, always-on-the-run personality, the doctors didn't think that was a good idea. If they could possibly save her sphincter, they would.

There was another treatment plan complication, too. Myra's cancer was a squamous cell carcinoma inside the colon wall. That was not the type of tumor typically found in the colon, so the doctors would have to use a different type of chemotherapy than normal.

So many possibilities, so many points of view. With a telephone call from one of the consulting doctors, Myra and Tim got an appointment with a prestigious specialist at UCLA. More information. More possibilities. More decisions.

To add to the confusion, everyone—friends, relatives, friends of friends, casual acquaintances—seemed to have an opinion on Myra's treatment. She tried to be polite and open-minded, even appreciative of everyone's concern. And anyway, someone really might have something important to share.

What to do?

A woman with whom Myra had worked got it into her head that if Myra so much as began a regimen of chemotherapy, she would die. This woman was a good friend of a doctor who had cured herself of cancer without using any chemo or radiation. The woman kept calling Myra and telling her, "You've *got* to talk to my friend!" Myra refused to answer the woman's calls. Then the woman's doctor friend started calling. Myra refused to answer her calls as well. Finally the doctor began faxing piles of material. When her friend called to see if she had gotten the information, Myra shouted, "I don't want to talk about this anymore! I don't want to hear about it anymore, not from you and not from your friend!" and hung up the phone.

Still, the "badgering" had some effect. Myra called the doctor and told him she was scared to death of going ahead with the chemotherapy because of people's dire warnings. "You come down here right now with your husband," he said. "I want to talk to both of you. Because we have a cancer here that we can stop. But if you don't do what needs to be done, I can't promise you anything."

Tim and Myra sat across the desk from the doctor. "Look," the doctor said. "You want alternative ideas? Here." And he handed them an assortment of books on alternative therapies. "If you are so far gone that there's nothing more we can do, I'll take you personally to any of these places. But we're not at that place yet. And right now, chemotherapy and radiation are your best shot. That's the bottom line."

In the wee hours of the next morning, Tim got up, went to his office, and got out the business plan he had prepared. Using the advice he had gleaned from the specialists and weaving in the best of what he and Myra had researched and read, he expanded the plan from a general approach to a specific and detailed blueprint for handling Myra's cancer. No more second-guessing. No more searching for a response when someone had a new miracle supplement to sell. No running from doctor to doctor, from treatment to treatment. From here on out, Tim and Myra would follow the plan.

Myra was blessed indeed. It's wonderful to have a capable, caring person to serve as your own personal case manager. Not everyone is so fortunate, however.

"I'm single," said 41-year-old Caroline, "and I'm sorry to say I'm not close to the few relatives I have. Just imagine going to the doctor for a routine checkup, being frightened into having a mole removed from your face, being informed that you have an aggressive melanoma that will require follow-up therapy with dicey results, and having no one to come home to lay it on. I have two really sweet cats, but they don't give much input in times like this. At first I thought I would just curl up on the couch and die. But I didn't. Instead, I discovered a wonderful thing about myself: I'm capable of doing a whole lot more than I ever thought I could! I was actually able to take charge and manage my own case. Who would have thought it?"

ASK THE RIGHT QUESTIONS

Fear and pain can make us scream out questions and demands for answers. Those quick fixes—are they too good to be true? Rumored escape hatches—do they really exist? It makes sense to put together a battle plan, but how can we do it properly?

Soberly and with wise counsel—that's how.

Yes, choosing the best treatment plan for your cancer certainly is a complex undertaking. That's because

- Cancer is not just one disease.
- Many varieties of drugs are available.
- Different drugs work better for different types of cancer.

- Different drugs work better for different people.
- The side effects of various treatments are not the same for everyone.
- Ongoing studies are constantly changing the face of cancer treatment.

The bottom line is that it's up to you to become informed. You can't depend upon anyone to give you all the information you need. You must ask. And ask. And ask. And ask some more. Keep on asking until you get an answer you can understand and that makes sense to you.

In addition to asking questions,

- Read the statistics.
- Get your hands on all the information you can about your type of cancer.
- Consider the advice and opinions of your doctors, family, and friends.

Now take all this information and look it over carefully. Consider each possibility. Weigh all your options. Pray for guidance. Wait upon the Lord. Ask others to pray with and for you.

Then make your choices.

Do you see what's happening here? You're refusing to be a victim and are insisting on being a participant.

Victims Say	Participants Say
I must	I choose
I'm helpless	I'm empowered
I should	I will
They won't let me	I choose not to
I can't	With God's help, I can!

Victims are helpless. Participants move forward in the power of God.

SIX RULES FOR TAKING CHARGE

"From the very beginning, I believed that the key to survival was finding out everything I could about the fairly rare type of brain cancer I had," said Justin. "One of the first things I learned was that cutting-edge research was going on right here in Chicago, not half an hour from my home. I pushed and pushed to get involved. I mean, I tried my best not to be obnoxious to my doctors, but my main concern was to know every treatment possibility I could so that I could make informed decisions. And if I became too sick to make decisions, I wanted my wife, Nancy, to be ready to take over for me. I wanted to be a nice guy, but if need be, I was prepared to fight tooth and nail. I wanted to do it, and I wanted to do it right."

Sounds awfully pushy, you say? Well, maybe, but it boggled my mind that my mother-in-law was willing to blindly submit to a surgeon who couldn't understand why she would balk at having her breast removed when she was just "an old woman." Why are so many people willing to walk blindly into one of the most important decisions of their lives? Perhaps because they don't know what else to do. Perhaps they don't understand that they do have choices. Perhaps it simply never occurs to them to make a proper plan they can use as a guide.

So how exactly do you go about making such a plan, and how can you be sure you are doing it properly? The following seven rules for taking charge will help as you create your own battle plan.

Rule 1: Choose medical care with which you can be comfortable.

It's important that you feel comfortable about the medical care you're receiving. Otherwise, you'll be plagued by worries and fears that can negatively affect your healing. Obviously, not all doctors are the same. Choose one who is a well-trained oncologist, experienced in dealing with your particular kind of cancer. The more experience the doctor has, the greater is his or her expertise. The more skilled, the more knowledgeable, the more experienced, the better.

At the very least you should be able to have a cordial relationship with the doctor. If you don't, it will be very difficult to talk freely, to ask questions, and to discuss your treatment together.

Oh, and one more thing. I love this quote from Jason Winters in *Killing Cancer:* "Find a doctor who believes God is greater than the medical associations, and you have found a jewel."[1]

Amen!

Rule 2: Don't go to the doctor's office alone.

The more important the subject, the more essential it is to have two pairs of ears listening. Myra had Tim. Justin had Nancy. It's nice to have a spouse—unless that spouse is so rattled that he or she not only doesn't absorb anything but also distracts you from listening as well. Or your spouse refuses to go ("Doctors' offices make me sick!"). Or you don't have a spouse.

Robert was in his last year of college when he was diagnosed with testicular cancer. He wasn't married, he lived across the country from his family, and his friends were, in his words, "freaked out" about his disease. "It sounds silly and cold," Robert said, "but in the end it was one of the counselors at the university who offered to go to my appointments with me. At first I said no. I mean, I didn't need babysitting or anything. But I was so wracked up and everything I missed half of what the doctor told me. So I took Mac up on his offer."

Four ears are better than two. Two brains are better than one. And a caring arm around the shoulder on the way out of the doctor's office is priceless.

Rule 3: Be a stickler for information.

For many cancers, a wide array of options and possible treatments is available. Each has its own advantages, disadvantages, risks, benefits, and potential side effects. The only way you can appreciate these distinctions is to take the time and effort to become aware of and to carefully consider each. Ask your doctor for information. Sure, your doctor is busy, but don't let him or her get away without giving you the answers you need. If you don't get them, ask again. Confused? Press for clarification.

Ask the doctor where you can get more information on your specific condition or on the suggested treatment. Ask if there are other patients with whom you might talk, those who have already been through a specific treatment. Ask such a person for advice and suggestions. (Many of the cancer survivors in this book—including Myra Mahoney—have made themselves available to other cancer patients who are facing the treatments they have already completed.)

Don't hesitate to get a second opinion—or a third, for that matter.

Rule 4: Refuse to be controlled by fear.

When Emily sat down to discuss a course of treatment for her breast cancer, all she could do was cry. She was only 13 when her own mother had died of the disease. Now she sobbed for her own young children who might well be motherless before they even reached an age of double digits.

Fear: for many cancer sufferers it is the predominant emotion. In fact, because of all the horror stories they have heard, many patients regard chemotherapy and radiation treatments with almost as much fear and dread as they have for the disease itself.

Yes, you're in a scary place. Yes, things are uncertain. But it's imperative that you force yourself to set your fear aside while you put your battle plan together. You must do it. Fear is a poor starting place for making such important decisions.

Rule 5: Keep up with cancer breakthroughs.

The good news is that many new breakthroughs in cancer treatment are occurring. Your challenge is to make sure you know about the ones that affect your type of cancer. For instance, solid tumors of the lung, prostate, breast, and colon share common targets that new experimental therapies are designed to attack. Emily, who suffered from breast cancer, searched these out and took advantage of them. Theo, who had lung cancer, likely could have benefited as well, but he never looked beyond his local hometown doctor, so he knew nothing about it. While targeted therapies are unlikely to replace standard chemotherapy, when combined with it, they may well offer a powerful new tool.

Sue Stewart's *Newsletter* online includes a resource directory with direct links to both medical sites and financial aid information. The National Cancer Institute is another great resource. The data is free and easy to navigate. If you want the latest research on your specific disease, you can access medical journals.[2]

Rule 6: Don't lose your perspective.

Let's face it: no matter what you do, you're not going to become an expert overnight. To be sure you're keeping things in their proper perspective,

- Take the information to your doctors and discuss it with them. Not everything you read will apply to you and your situation.
- Ask questions, but don't drive your doctor crazy.
- Cooperate, but don't surrender.
- Be your own case manager, but don't run it into the ground.

COMPLEMENTARY TREATMENTS

So what's worth trying? Everything. Chemotherapy and radiation. Investigating the latest research. Eating well and exercising. Alternatives—within appropriate parameters. Prayer, of course, is indispensable. And ask others to pray. Do it all.

Latest Research

Thirty-six-year-old Jen was in the prime of her life when she was informed that she had chronic myeloid leukemia, an especially deadly form of blood cancer. "I'm sorry, but you only have months to live," her doctor told her. "You had best get your affairs in order."

Her affairs? Jen's main affair was the mother-daughter soccer team she and her 10-year-old daughter LeeAnn had played on together for three years. Even when Jen was too weary to run more than a couple of yards, she struggled out onto the field, determined to continue with those games. But now, her eyes clouded with tears, she dutifully sat down and started making a list of who would get what:

Grandmother Davidson's china—sister Elizabeth

Grandmother Quinn's quilt—daughter LeeAnn

Great-grandfather Quinn's family Bible—Ryan (He's only 5. Will he even care?)

Jewelry—LeeAnn (Maybe save something for Ryan's wife . . . wife?)

My clothes—wouldn't fit Elizabeth. Just give them to charity.
My library of books?—

All the while Jen was bravely enduring treatments that no one had the least hope would cure her. But guess what. That was seven years ago. No, the treatments didn't cure her, but they did keep her alive until she could be admitted to studies of the drug Gleevec, which was approved by the United States Food and Drug Administration in 2001. This new drug, based on the principle of molecular targeting—that is, killing leukemia cells while leaving normal white cells alone—worked wonders. Today Jen is in complete remission.

Eight years ago there were 124 medicines in the research pipeline being tested as potential anticancer agents. As I write this, there are 402. By the time you read this book, there are sure to be even more. Some are traditional, but many are a whole new breed. To see what's out there, you can check the Pharmaceutical Research and Manufacturers of America web site at <www.phrma.org>.

Complementary Alternative Products

A while back, actress and fitness advocate Suzanne Somers announced she had breast cancer and that instead of traditional chemotherapy treatments, she was choosing to inject herself with Iscador, a remedy made of mistletoe extract. Cancer experts shuddered. Imagine the message that sent to other cancer sufferers. Rita Mehta, assistant clinical professor of medicine at the University of California, Irvine, and an oncologist and hematologist, said of Somers, "She said she made an informed choice, but in my opinion it wasn't informed enough. I'm not saying Iscador will never work against breast cancer, but we don't have the evidence right now that shows it works."

Gleevec? Iscador? Neither means a lot to most of us. But to learn the distinction can mean the difference between life and death.

Certainly I'm not suggesting you turn your back on all alternative therapies. It makes no sense to overlook the legitimate ones that really *can* help you, because so many are pseudo-medical fakes. While some alternatives have shown some benefits, others are downright dangerous. By far, the best approach is to resist abandoning the traditional treatments, even though you fear the side effects. To do so is to risk your life. Far better, according to Barrie Cassileth, who runs the complementary-care program at New York City's Memorial Sloan-Kettering Cancer Center, is to look toward "complementary treatments"—those that are used along with, rather than instead of, mainstream care. They can be herbs or natural products that enhance the immune system, such as garlic.

Larry Burkett in his book *Hope When It Hurts* suggests three criteria for alternative therapies:

1. *Scientific merit*. Burkett insists that any alternative therapy have some scientific proof, based on repeatable, verifiable data. Many alternatives admonish participants that they must have "blind faith"—not in God, but in the treatment itself.

2. *No harm*. The treatment chosen should pose no further harm to one's body. It has to be nontoxic. Many times where alternatives are concerned, you're dealing with people who are not thoroughly trained in medicine.

3. *Referrals*. Burkett says it's extremely important to talk to people who have taken the treatment and survived. Don't depend on anecdotal or testimonial data alone.[3]

A Time to Gather, a Time to Stop Gathering

In order to know your options, you need to gather information. But the time comes when you must stop gathering. As my first husband, Larry's, health deteriorated, I followed up on lead after lead after lead. Finally a dear brother in our church, a neurosurgeon by the name of Paul, telephoned me and said, "Kay, please listen to me. You must not devote your life to looking for an answer that doesn't exist. It's time to look at what is and deal with it. If you don't, you're going to drive both yourself and Larry crazy, and you'll go broke in the process."

I didn't want to hear what Paul had to say, but it was the truth.

You can continue gathering information until the end of time. As one doctor said, "Don't get 2-second opinions in an effort to find the answer you're looking for. People die doing that."

So how do you know when it's time to stop looking? Ask yourself the following 12 questions, and let the answers help guide you:

1. Do I know all I need to know in order to make the best possible decision?
2. Do I understand the meaning of the information I have gathered?
3. Do I trust my doctor?
4. Do I know and understand what the alternatives are?
5. Am I praying, and are others praying, for God's leading in my decisions?
6. How can I get the maximum benefit from conventional cancer treatments while minimizing the risk as well as my own discomfort?
7. How might I integrate complementary and alternative therapies into my treatment?
8. Can I talk to my doctor about the complementary and alternative treatments I'm considering?
9. What particular attention should I be paying to my diet?
10. What vitamins, minerals, and supplements should I be taking?

11. How much should I exercise, or should I just rest as much as I can right now?

12. What can I do to minimize the side effects of my cancer treatment?

In any treatments and therapies, you'll find a trade-off between what you can gain and the price you'll have to pay. Is the benefit worth the cost? That final decision is up to you.

"I made a decision to have a mastectomy even though my doctor said it was not necessary," Marlene said. "The thing is, my mother, my grandmother, and my great-grandmother all died of breast cancer. I'm 58 years old, and this is my second bout with the disease. I'll be the first to acknowledge that this radical surgery is not for everyone. But I weighed all my options and decided this is the choice I can best live with. If my cancer comes back again, I'll know I did everything I could. I'll never have to look back and say, 'I wish I had done more.'"

As you make your battle plan, remember one final thought: The greatest battles you—like any of us—will ever fight are those within yourself. When the pressure builds up beyond endurance, and, despite yourself, you cry out against God or run and hide in despair, then know that it's time for you to turn your battle plan over to Him. For He alone can give you the strength to see it through. And at that moment, when you open your mouth to cry out, *Help me, Lord!* He'll be answering, *My child, I'm helping you already.*

Before they call I will answer;
while they are still speaking I will hear *(Isa. 65:24).*

6

A Declaration of Dependence

"My life is full, fulfilling, and filled with adventure," Nick wrote in his Christmas letter. "I couldn't be happier!" No wonder! At 46, Nick was at the height of his professional career. His wife, Donna, was an active member of the school board and was making a positive difference in their community. Their teenage sons, Ben and Josh, were everything a mother and father could wish for, and their "little miracle," five-year-old Suzie, was her daddy's pride and joy.

Early in January, as Nick and Suzie were working together on the forest mural they were painting on the dining room wall, Suzie said, "Daddy, how come you cough all the time?"

"I don't know," Nick said. "Just something in my throat, I guess."

"But it never gets out of your throat," Suzie said.

"Yeah," Nick agreed. "Guess I'll call the doctor. Maybe there's a bug in there."

The "bug" turned out to be esophageal cancer.

Nick later recalled, "I walked away from that diagnosis with iron determination. I *had* to conquer that cancer! I had to do it for Donna, and for Ben and Josh. But most of all, I had to do it for Suzie."

INDEPENDENCE?

Like Nick, most of us tend to approach such a diagnosis with the belief that we have no resources other than what we can drum up in ourselves and that those just *have* to be enough.

Vulnerable? No way! We must be in control!

But independence is all an illusion. If we didn't know it before, we certainly know it now. Independence is more than impossible. It isn't even desirable. In a study at Duke University, researchers found that older adults who rarely prayed had a 50 percent greater risk of dying than those who prayed once a month or more.

This would not surprise the apostle Paul one bit. Look at what he wrote in his second letter to the church at Corinth about his time in Asia: "We had the sentence of death in ourselves, that we should not trust in ourselves but in God who raises the dead, who delivered us from so great a death, and does deliver us; in whom we trust that He will still deliver us" (2 Cor. 1:9-10, NKJV). In Asia the battered apostle was pushed to the absolute edge of his endurance. And then he was nudged a bit farther. He was right on the line between life and death. Talk about being desperate beyond your own strength!

Do you notice verse 9? Paul puts his finger on another reason for our times of sorrow: that we might come to a complete end of ourselves and learn the power of total dependence.

"It didn't take me long to realize that I didn't want to be independent," Nick said, "and I didn't care who knew it. Then and there I made my official declaration of dependence on God!"

GOD WORKING IN ME

That's not to say that we throw in the towel and say, "Oh, whatever, God!" No, it's up to us to keep on keeping on. The key here is in Phil. 2:13—"It is God who works in you to will and to act according to his good purpose."

Such a declaration of dependence frees us to do all we can do, to keep a positive attitude, to maintain a position of unflagging hope, and yet to relinquish the responsibility to God. Only then can we come to where we can honestly give thanks in every tribulation.

Give Thanks

We *can* learn to thank God, because it's He who gives us strength when we feel so weak and helpless. That's why Paul could say, "I take pleasure in infirmities . . . in distresses, for Christ's sake" (2 Cor. 12:10, NKJV). And as believers in Jesus Christ and in the truth of His Word, we can be grateful that through even this experience, God is accomplishing what is best for us. Even through our suffering, He's working for our good (Rom. 8:28).

"I lay on the couch and look at the half-painted mural," Nick said. "Suzie caresses my head and says, 'Daddy, I wish we could paint.' I tell her I wish we could, too, but I'm too tired. I'm just too tired."

Strength in Dependence

Too tired. Too tired. You know how that feels, don't you? You've been there. But here's another advantage of the "declaration of dependence": it brings *strength.*

Let me tell you about strength. Better yet, let the ancient prophet Isaiah tell you:

Do you not know? Have you not heard?
The Everlasting God, the LORD, the Creator
     of the ends of the earth
Does not become weary or tired.
His understanding is inscrutable.
He gives strength to the weary,
And to him who lacks might He increases power.
Though youths grow weary and tired,
And vigorous young men stumble badly,
Yet those who wait for the LORD
Will gain new strength;
They will mount up with wings like eagles,
They will run and not get tired,
They will walk and not become weary *(40:28-31, NASB).*

Ahh—to soar on wings like eagles and never grow tired! To paint your mural and not grow weary! To run, to walk, to work, to play! Wait on the Lord. Just wait on Him.

All of us will sooner or later be called on to trust God as we endure some great challenge of sickness, grief, or great disappointment. And it is then that we must *walk by faith, not by sight* (2 Cor. 5:7). This is your time.

It's your time to
- Learn to be a taker rather than a giver.
- Lean on your support system.
- Call on your friends and family.
- Talk and pray with other believers.
- Let your pastor and your church know practical ways in which they can be of help to you.
- Graciously accept what's offered to you.

Unlimited Resources

"The background on our mural is a sunny gold," Nick says. "I sketched in an autumn forest scene with a stream running through it. There are trees of many different species, ferns and other plants, birds in the trees, and small animals on the ground. Everywhere you look is an unexpected surprise. On the lower quarter I outlined everything and marked it with the appropriate color so that Suzie could do the actual painting."

After a pause he continues, "My cancer is in remission, and my strength is much improved. I'm pleased to say that Suzie and I are 90 percent finished with our mural. In fact, we would be completely done if one or the other of us didn't keep thinking of something else to hide away in the golden forest!"

I had the privilege of seeing Nick and Suzie's magnificent mural in all its almost-completed grandeur. As I looked at the "before" and "after" photos, I couldn't help but think of the transformation that takes place in our lives when God applies His full array of resources. On our own, we're like Nick's original bare beige wall, meager and puny with precious little to commend us. But then the Master goes to work with His full palette—magnificent shades of wisdom, peace, patience, the will to endure. And, oh, what a glorious masterpiece He produces!

Don't underestimate the extent of the resources God brings to bear on your life. Remember how Heb. 12:1 tells us of the "great cloud of witnesses" that surrounds us? Within this vast cloud are those biblical heroes who have so inspired us—men and women like Abraham and David and Noah and Esther and Deborah and Paul and Peter and so many, many more. They trusted God in their afflictions and persecution and in suffering we can't begin to imagine. Their words give us a language of grief. Their faithfulness and endurance give us perspective. Their triumph gives us hope.

Just imagine! The Master Artist is at work. His resources are all there at your disposal. And all the while that huge cloud of witnesses is cheering you on. "Don't give up!" they're calling out. "It will be worth it all! Believe us—we know! We've been there, and now we're on the other side. Hang on, Christian! Hang on! Keep up the good work!"

THE GRACE OF GOD

A declaration of dependence? It really makes sense to relinquish control when you realize that you never were in control in the first place!

When we finally quit fighting for independence, one of the easiest and the hardest things to do is to pray. It's easiest because we so want God to take over. It's hardest because we just can't seem to find the words. God knew we would have that problem. Look what He led the apostle Paul to write in Rom. 8:26—"We do not know what we ought to pray for, but the Spirit himself intercedes for us with groans that words cannot express." When you pray in the Spirit, God *always* hears, and He *always* understands. And He *always* moves mightily!

Want to know what else comes with dependence? Confidence. Total, all-encompassing, everlasting confidence! In Rom. 8:35, 37-39 we read,

Who will separate us from the love of Christ? Will tribulation, or distress, or persecution, or famine, or nakedness, or peril, or sword? . . . But in all these things we overwhelmingly conquer through Him who loved us. For I am convinced that neither death, nor life, nor angels, nor principalities, nor things present, nor things to come, nor powers, nor height, nor depth, nor any other created thing, will be able to separate us from the love of God, which is in Christ Jesus our Lord (NASB).

Cancer does not separate us from God's love. He is always with us, even in the midst of suffering and even in the midst of cancer. This we can depend on. Now that's what I call *blessed dependence!*

1
THE CHALLENGE OF ENDURANCE

When Jen began her journey through leukemia, she determined to keep a journal, recording each step of the way. And she did. Through the innumerable treatments—chemotherapy, radiation, bone marrow transplant—through the loneliness of isolation day after day after day, including Christmas, Thanksgiving, and her daughter's birthday. Through it all, Jen faithfully kept her journal. But finally, one week all she could manage to write was *Dear God, I can't face another day!*

There are times when it's too much. It's just too much.

I've never before considered the ability to go potty as a blessing, but I do now, Jen wrote one day.

On another: *Dr. Grenaldi told me I would lose my hair very rapidly, probably within a week. Immediately handfuls of my beautiful long, chestnut hair started falling out. Seven days later I was completely bald. Talk about traumatic and depressing!*

No matter how surrounded you are, dear one, no matter how supported by caring people, ultimately you're the one who has to face your cancer. It's you who endures those treatments. It's you who confronts the nagging fear of death.

"You know what was especially hard for me?" asked Caroline, a 41-year-old model whose "signature mole" turned out to be melanoma. "It was feeling physically fine even with cancer running around in my body. Then I submitted to treatment that made me feel truly horrendous. By the time I felt better again, it was time for another dose, and the whole routine started over again. It was terrifying to submit my seemingly well body to crippling rounds of poison."

Unlike Caroline, Jen didn't feel so great before her leukemia was diagnosed. Still, she, too, struggled with the demands of enduring. *I'M SO TIRED OF THIS!* She wrote in angry letters across one entire page. *HOW LONG IS THIS GOING TO GO ON?*

Doctors, nurses, and medical technicians, the very ones who are fighting alongside you, are not always emotionally as caring as they should be. Many times they get so caught up in their own busy schedules that they forget they're dealing with living, breathing people whose struggles go much deeper than a battle of cells and blood counts and lab tests.

For Keith, the diagnosis of liver cancer was too staggering. The odds the doctor gave him were too heavily stacked against him. The swirling stories of the terrors of chemotherapy and radiation were too horrifying. The whispered warnings about medical conspiracies were too convincing. Despite his wife's attempts to buck him up and be encouraging, Keith lost faith in mainstream medical approaches. Lured on by strangers' extravagant promises and outsized tales of success, Keith rapidly went through their life savings. It cost a lot to run from the United States to Mexico and the Bahamas in his desperate search for a cure. He tried endless diet therapies and endured cleansing programs, coffee enemas, and high-dose intravenous vitamin infusions. Shark cartilage, Asian teas, mistletoe extract—anything that offered even a tiny ray of hope was fair game.

Thinking back on that time, Keith's wife, Linda, said, "It was so sad to watch. With the horrendous cost of it all, we were literally plummeting toward bankruptcy. But all Keith could see was the hopelessness of what the medical establishment had to offer him, and the hope—however farfetched and self-serving—these other people were extending."

THE HILL TOO STEEP

When you look at your own battle plan and see what you have to go through, you may well cry, "I can't do it! That hill is just too high and too steep for me to climb. Maybe someone in really good shape could make it, someone young and healthy, someone who has spent long hours at the gym, maybe—someone who's not me."

Funny thing about hills, though. Many people perceive them to be steeper than they really are, especially if they're tired or burdened down with a heavy load. Thinking about what lies before us exhausts and overwhelms us before we even start.

Jen understood that. Lying in her bed in isolation awaiting a bone marrow transplant that may or may not work, she found it an effort just to hold her arm up and write. But she did. And her journal speaks of her frustration and exhaustion: *Sick . . . alone . . . scared. Dear God, when will it end? How will it end? Can I ever possibly hang on that long?*

I must not think about it. If I do, it will overwhelm me, and I won't be able to face one more tomorrow.

Too hard. Too painful. Too long a road. Too steep a hill.

What are you fixing your sights on? The top of the hill? The mountaintop? The tip of a distant peak shrouded in impenetrable clouds? If so, you may perceive the hill as far, far too steep, the journey as unendurable.

"I started my chemotherapy full of positive feelings," Marlene recalled of her latest bout with breast cancer. "Then my hair started to fall out. I had my sister shave my head that weekend, and for the first time I started to bawl. Having no hair was worse than having no breasts, because people knew by looking at me that something was very wrong. Everyone, even strangers, felt sorry for me. I got a wig, but it was so annoying that I started wearing scarves and hats. (Man, am I sick of hats!) You know what wore me down even more than the nausea and weariness? How some people were so uncomfortable around me. It was as if I was a constant reminder that they, too, were vulnerable."

Marlene, who all her life had been independent, had always felt more comfortable doing for someone else than being done for. Now she felt completely defeated by her vulnerability. Stuck with a problem she couldn't solve, she dragged herself up the hill in too much pain to care whether she made the next step or not.

Pain Control

It's hard to keep your emotions under control and your journey toward recovery focused when your pain is out of control. Determine right here and now not to put up with more pain than you have to. Let your doctor know just how much pain you're experiencing. Better to err on the side of whining, I always say, than on trying to be too stoic and then ending up suffering needlessly.

You say, quit complaining when nothing can be done about the pain? Listen to this consensus statement from the National Cancer Institute: "In approximately 90% of patients, cancer pain can be controlled through relatively simple means."[1]

"But I don't want to become addicted to pain medication," you may say.

Don't worry. It almost never happens. And if by some strange chance it did, it could be taken care of at a later date. Right now, concern yourself with improving your battle readiness by controlling the pain. Suffering in silence doesn't show bravery or faith or anything else positive.

ONE STEP AT A TIME

There are times to lift your eyes up to the hills, and there are times to focus them firmly on that one step you can manage right now. This is not the time for long-range sight-setting. No, it's the time for here-and-now foot-planting. You took yesterday's step yesterday. Good for you! Today keep your sights firmly focused on today's step.

Tomorrow's step? Don't worry about it, let alone next week's or next month's. Here are some ideas to help you take today's step today:

Stay Active

1. Do something! Choose activities (or just one activity) that are comfortable, accessible to you, and that you really like to do.
2. Continue with exercises that help maintain or increase your energy during your treatment and afterward. (Don't think strenuous or muscle-building here. There was a point in Marlene's treatment where she was so tired that her exercise of choice was rolling over and over in bed!)
3. Cardiovascular activity can boost your spirit, help you to be less tired, prop up your immune system, and speed up your recovery. "As soon as I could get out of bed I started walking," Marlene said, "first around the house, then around the yard, then around the neighborhood." Actually, walking is a good way to start. Begin with 5-10 minutes, once or twice every other day. Gradually increase at a comfortable pace so that you can walk up to 30-45 minutes a day. But if 10-15 minutes is what feels most comfortable, stay at that level. Remember: this is today's step you're taking.
4. On days when you feel good, do more things and get more exercise. On days when you feel tired, rest more or select an easier activity. Caroline's favorite "draggy day" activity was to stretch gently to music.
5. Check to see if there are exercise programs that support cancer survivors in your community. (Here in Santa Barbara, California, for instance, we have a facility called Cancer Wellness.) If not, find an exercise partner who will keep you encouraged and motivated. (Every day, rain or shine, Theo and his wife walk their dogs in the park. The motivator? "My dogs!

They have to be walked. As long as I have my 'gold-
ies' I will take my daily walks.")

Be You!

"I gave up my wig after the first couple scratchy days,"
Marlene recalled of her last round of treatment. "In time I
gave up my hats, too. I really do look awful in hats! Yes, I
got funny looks and embarrassing stares, what with my
bald head and all. But who cared? With what I was going
through, with all I had gone through already, what were a
few stares?"

Marlene doesn't let anyone else tell her who and what
she ought to be. She would love to know Leslie Mouton,
an attractive, young San Antonio news anchorwoman.

Let me tell you about Leslie: Makeup done to a "T" and
finished off with shiny red lipstick. A snappy outfit and
gold earrings that glittered in the bright television studio
lights. On that particular evening, just like most every
weekday evening, Leslie perched atop her swivel chair and
smiled into the camera.

But wait, something was not the same that particular
evening. Thirty-six-year-old Leslie was completely bald!
Yes, viewers may have been shocked to see her shiny pate,
but few asked why. Certainly not if they tuned in to KSAT-
TV even semi-regularly. This was Leslie's third report on
her very personal battle with cancer. The first night viewers saw her on the operating table. On the second they
bore witness to the tears that filled her eyes as the first
chemotherapy drugs were pumped into her chest. And
now they saw her unashamedly anchoring the news without her wig.

A tear-jerker ploy during ratings sweeps week?

"Not at all!" insisted Leslie, who describes herself as a
born-again Christian. "This was God's timing, not mine."

God had put Leslie Mouton where she was, just at that
time, "for such a time as this."

Allow yourself to be who you are. Don't be controlled

by pressure from those around you. This is your life. God has put you here right now. And He has a sovereign reason for it.

Cope However You Can

The challenge of endurance is to cope. One person's coping methods may not work for another person, but hey—it's all worth a try!

"Give yourself time to cry, because it's healthy," Jen advises, "but then stop crying and move on. Read positive stories and magazine articles. Watch upbeat TV shows and movies. You've got plenty of time to deal with the heavy side of life. This isn't it."

Jen can speak about the challenges of endurance. She had such a heavy dose of both radiation and chemotherapy concurrently that she developed a rash that turned her entire body deep red and purple. "My skin was burned from the inside out. Finally it turned a leathery brown. The outside layer of my mouth and gastrointestinal tract blistered and peeled off. I was bald, my eyes were bloody, my body was covered with ugly splotches—my skin was falling off my bones. LeeAnn and Ryan weren't even allowed to see me. I looked so awful that the doctor and my husband felt they would be too traumatized."

And yet Jen coped. How?

"Only one way," Jen says emphatically. "Only by God's grace. Only because I knew without a shadow of a doubt that I was in His hands and therefore, in any situation life presented me, there was hope. I recited my favorite Scripture verse over and over and over again: 'Do not fear, for I am with you; do not be dismayed, for I am your God. I will strengthen you and help you; I will uphold you with my righteous right hand' [Isa. 41:10]."

Make Fun Happen

In 1964 a man by the name of Norman Cousins fell ill with a rare and incurable disease that degenerates the connective tissue throughout the body. When he was told nothing could be done to save his life, he checked himself out of the hospital and into a hotel across the street. Determined to put himself into a more positive frame of mind, he played funny movies, read funny books, and did anything he could think of to make himself laugh nonstop. His frame of mind did change, but an even more interesting thing happened. He found that all that laughter was actually blocking the terrible pain he had been suffering. To everyone's amazement, Cousins not only didn't die, but he actually recovered. He told everyone what had happened to him and then wrote a book about it. The rest, as they say, is history. Today laughter is an important part of many cancer treatment approaches.

In fact, scientists now believe there's an actual physical link between chemicals manufactured in the brain (neurochemicals) and those in the rest of the body, including the immune system. Though there's a lot that's still not understood, it certainly seems that laughter can be valuable in fighting cancer. It certainly can't hurt! Why not take a break and have a little fun?

"I personally am a great believer in laughing my way to better and better health," Justin said with his usual conviction. "My personal favorites are *Calvin and Hobbs*, old television reruns like *The Andy Griffith Show,* and good old slapstick movies. There's nothing like belly laughs to relieve stress and begin to change body chemistry, and I heartily recommend it."

Wise King Solomon, were he still around, just might agree. "A cheerful heart is good medicine," he wrote, "but a crushed spirit dries up the bones" (Prov. 17:22).

ENDURANCE IS A TEAM ACTIVITY

You don't have to have someone else with you to help you endure. It's possible to do it alone. But it sure is a lot easier and a whole lot less painful if you take it on as a team activity. Just listen to what some who have been there have to say:

"When I got out of the hospital, my family teamwork carried me through," said Jen. "My husband and mother and children changed their diet to match what I needed to eat. If I was on salads, we all ate salads. If I gave up meat, we all gave it up. When sugar went from my diet, it disappeared from the house. That teamwork meant so much to me!"

"I almost blew it," Justin admitted. "I didn't want people to feel sorry for me, so for a long time I wouldn't reach out to anyone, not even to those who loved me the most. Yet they were the very ones who could have been my lifeline. The thing was, I just couldn't comprehend how difficult this was for the ones closest to me, too. Every relationship—with my wife, my son, my daughter, my mother, my brother—every one of them was undergoing a huge strain."

"I don't have any family to speak of," said Caroline. "So just who was my endurance team supposed to be?"

Good question. Fair question.

Actually, Caroline's answer knocked at the door in the person of a neighbor by the name of Annette. "She really cared about me," Caroline said. "She came to my house every day and made me get out of bed and put my clothes on. She brought me homemade soup when I preferred not to eat. She made me walk when I longed to just lie in bed. When everyone else had written me off, Annette treated me like I was a living, breathing person with a future worth preserving. She asked me how I was doing and waited for an answer. How could she know how much I longed to have someone ask? I needed to vent, to yell, to cry. And I needed to have someone listen and care. Annette cared, and she loved me back to health."

"People prayed for me," Nick said. "Whenever someone said, 'I'm praying for you,' I said, 'Great—I'm holding you to it!' And I wrote down that person's name. I felt those prayers, and I truly believe I'm here today because of them."

By faith you will climb that hill one step at a time.

THE IRRITANT OF GREAT PRICE

Two years ago my husband Dan's work required him to do quite a bit of traveling throughout Asia. While there, he started a modest collection of pearls for me. The first was a necklace of standard creamy white pearls—the first real gems I had ever owned. Next he delighted me with a strand of iridescent coral pearls. Then came earrings the color of rich antique rose. And then my favorite: a necklace of the most magnificent pearls in hues of purples and plums. Dan told me that the next time he goes to Asia he wants to get me a strand of silver-gray pearls. Fascinated by the endless hues and varieties—each pearl lustrous and unique—we got a book and read about how the beautiful precious stones are formed.

A grain of sand lodges in the tender flesh of an oyster and becomes a distressing irritation. Unable to get rid of it yet unable to live with the pain, the oyster patiently covers the tormenting irritant with layer after layer of a milky secretion. In time that irritation becomes smooth and acceptable. In the process, it becomes a precious jewel. Pearls, you see, are produced by overcoming great pain and destruction.

God, too, patiently lays layer after layer of grace upon your unacceptable pain until that distressing irritation in your life becomes a precious gem to His glory. A pearl of great price.

8
THE POWER SOURCE

"My mouth was completely covered with horrible sores," Myra said of her massive chemotherapy/radiation barrage. "I was in such awful shape people would just look at me and cry. They would come over to bring us dinner, intending to stay awhile to cheer me up and pray with me, but when they saw me, they could do nothing but stand and weep. And I knew perfectly well what was going through their minds. They just knew I was going to die."

Your power is drained away. You don't want to succumb to hopelessness and despair, but you simply cannot summon the strength to grasp a brighter, more positive perspective.

We struggle to see what's before us, to reach out and grasp, then to cling to something tangible. But that's not how it is, is it?

And why should we be surprised? 2 Cor. 4:18 tells us, "We do not look at the things which are seen, but at the things which are not seen. For the things which are seen are temporary, but the things which are not seen are eternal" (NKJV).

Praise God!

CONSERVE YOUR POWER

Some of the things that drain your power need to be set aside. Relinquish to God everything that's a burden to you and anything that causes you anguish. For Myra, a huge power drain was her son's difficult and selfish behavior. For Nick it was the loss of his rich baritone singing voice. For Jen it was the Saturday afternoon mother-daughter soccer tournaments with LeeAnn. For Robert it was his university studies; he just couldn't keep up the demanding schedule. For Justin it was driving. The onset of seizures made it too dangerous, yet with his driver's license went the last vestige of independence.

"God whispers to us in our pleasures," C. S. Lewis wrote, "but shouts in our pain." The Lord God is the source of all power. That's always true. But now at this time He's shouting it so loudly, how can we fail to hear?

Stones of Remembrance

Forty years had passed since the Israelites left Egypt. It had been 40 years of frustrated wandering in the wilderness, 40 years of eating manna and quail, manna and quail, and still more manna and quail. Now the people were ready to cross the Jordan River and step into the Promised Land. Now, at long last, they were home.

But there was just one problem. It was the rainy season, and the Jordan was flooding its banks. There was no way the army and a million-plus people and all their warring and living stuff were ever going to make it across.

Enter Joshua. Speaking the words the Lord had given to him, he announced to the people,

> Come here and listen to the words of the LORD your God. This is how you will know that the living God is among you. . . . See, the ark of the covenant of the Lord of all the earth will go into the Jordan ahead of you. Now then, choose twelve men from the tribes of Israel, one from each tribe. And as soon as the priests who carry the ark of the LORD—the Lord of all the earth—set foot in the Jordan, its waters flowing downstream will be cut off and stand up in a heap (3:9-13).

And that's just what happened. The waters stood in a heap while all the people of Israel—men, women, and children, followed by goats and sheep and oxen, carts and tents and all the accumulations of 40 years—passed through on dry ground to the other side. When everyone and everything was safely across, Joshua called together the twelve men he had appointed, one from each tribe, and told them,

> Go over before the ark of the LORD your God into the middle of the Jordan. Each of you is to take up a stone on his shoulder, according to the number of the

tribes of the Israelites, to serve as a sign among you. In the future, when your children ask you, "What do these stones mean?" tell them that the flow of the Jordan was cut off before the ark of the covenant of the LORD. When it crossed the Jordan, the waters of the Jordan were cut off. These stones are to be a memorial to the people of Israel forever *(4:5-7)*.

These were stones of remembrance. I have stones of remembrance of my own. They came out of the ashes of my house after it was destroyed by fire. After I despaired of ever finding anything from my life before that devastation, my foot hit against something buried deep in the rubble. I reached down and picked up something hard and irregularly shaped, then blew off the thick coat of ashes that covered it. It looked like a piece of modern sculpture. Its base was formed by a set of turkey-shaped salt-and-pepper shakers, forever molded beak to beak by the crystal goblets that had melted over them. The turkeys had been a gift from my sixth-grade teacher who had always had such great faith in me and my potential. On top of the turkeys was the melted base of a silver candlestick, a wedding gift. To one side were the melted remains of my grandmother's milk glass sugar bowl, and on the other side was the delicate china cup I bought on our honeymoon. Balanced on one side was my daughter Lisa's baby spoon and fork, and on the other was my son Eric's long-handled baby feeding spoon. The entire piece was cemented together and glazed with crystal.

It was a summary of our family's life together before the fire. Before my first husband Larry's death. Before Lisa and Eric went away to college and then on into adult life. Before my memories of that life began to fade. It was my stone of remembrance.

For the next year and a half, until our home was rebuilt, we moved from place to place. Wherever we went, I carried my stone of remembrance with me and always put it in a prominent place. My kids would say, "Oh, Mom, are you going to put that on the mantle in this house too?" And I would say, "You bet your life I am!"

The apostle Paul, writing under inspiration from the Holy Spirit, wrote in Phil. 4:8, "Whatever is true, whatever is noble, whatever is right, whatever is pure, whatever is lovely, whatever is admirable—if anything is excellent or praiseworthy—think about such things."

When our stones of remembrance are piled right where they constantly stare us in the face, where they're in our pathway so that we have to take care not to trip over them, we cannot help but remember the deep valleys and the winding mountain trails over which God has safely led us.

"An incredible walk of faith went on in my house all through the difficult time of my cancer treatments," Myra said. "People were there at our house prodding and pulling and forcing me onward. We were well aware that we were the focus of prayer requests, and notes of love and encouragement poured in."

Tim's mother, who was not a believer, was a devoted caregiver for Myra. She flew to Santa Barbara from Tucson, Arizona, and got a hotel close to the Mahoneys' house. Each morning she arrived at Tim and Myra's house in time to drive the kids to school, and she stayed all day. She cleaned, did laundry, wrote thank-you notes, cared for Myra, and chauffeured the boys where they needed to go. After the dinner dishes were done, she said goodnight and went to her hotel.

But all day long she was with Myra. Nothing was lost on her. She would stick her head into Myra's room and see her typing full-speed on her laptop computer. "Would you please get off that computer?" she would insist kindly but firmly. "You're using up too much of your energy."

Obediently, Myra would scrunch down in bed and type more slowly. "Is this good enough, Mom?" she'd ask, then quickly explain, "I have to E-mail my prayer list. I need to have people pray for me."

Tim's mother observed memorial stones everywhere. She saw that, as sick as Myra was, she was able to make it to the Bible study fellowship every single week. And Tim's mother was there the day Myra got a card from a prayer warrior friend who wrote,

As I was praying for you this morning, the Lord gave me this verse from Isa. 43:2: "I will take you through the waters and you will not be overcome, I will take you through the fire and you will not be burned."

"Hey!" Myra exclaimed. "I had that verse in Bible study this week!"

"But, Myra, Dear," Tim's mother said, "look at you. Your lips are burned raw. You can't sit down without all those creams and pain medications from the doctor. Myra, you *have* been burned!"

"But, Mom," Myra told her mother-in-law, "I've walked through the fire and I haven't been burned *up*! I wasn't consumed!"

Mountains of Power

So what would your piled-up stones of remembrance have to do with the Power Source? Well, they would cause you to plug in to Him and, just at the time when you're so prone to forget, to remember how helpless you are on your own and how limitless the resources of your Power Source. All you need to do is

- Pile your stones of remembrance high.
- Make many, many piles.
- Put the piles in such prominent places that you're always running into them.
- Place them in locations where other people will see them and ask, "What's this?" Then you can answer, "I'm so glad you asked! Let me tell you what God did for me!"

When you fall into despair, or when you're at a loss for words to help another despairing soul, you'll stumble across your piled-up proof of past times when God proved his faithfulness and power. If He did it then, surely you can trust Him to do it now.

Today a major stone of remembrance in the Mahoneys' life is the way God worked in Tim's mother. She watched as Myra plugged into the Power Source again and again. She saw Him at work in Tim, making strength out of his weakness. And she saw Him in the prayer and words and deeds of their brothers and sisters in Christ. At the Mahoneys' home she repeatedly saw Jesus Christ at work through His people.

Power to . . .

At the turn of the millennium, the African nation of Mozambique was ravaged by horrendous floods. People frantically clambered up trees, climbing as high as they could to escape the rising waters. In one tree a pastor and 16 other people clung tightly to the highest branches, knowing their lives depended on their ability to hang on. As the hours dragged on and no rescuers came, the increasingly exhausted people begged, "Pastor, preach to us. It will help us stay awake." The preacher was also weary beyond endurance, but the mosquitoes were biting him so badly he couldn't possibly fall asleep. And so he preached. And he preached. And he preached. It was almost two full days before the exhausted group was rescued. Every exposed inch of the poor preacher was covered with mosquito bites; they had even bitten through his clothes! You know what he said of the ordeal? He said, "I thank God for those mosquitoes, because they stopped me from falling asleep. If I had fallen asleep, then others would have fallen asleep. And if we had fallen asleep, then one by one we would have been carried off by the water."

Thank God in all things.

The mystery of suffering is a Christian paradox. How do we reconcile suffering with triumphant victory? I don't have an easy answer. Yet Christ has assured us, "I have overcome the world." And I've seen God prove himself faithful and true too many times to doubt Him.

In my darkest time, I made myself a little sign and taped it on the bathroom mirror so that I could see it first thing every morning and last thing before I went to bed at night. It read,

EVEN WHEN YOU HIT BOTTOM
YOU STILL HAVE A ROCK TO STAND ON!
That Rock—the Lord God—is your Power Source!

9
SPIRITUAL QUESTIONS, SCRIPTURAL ANCHORS

Every day when the sun sinks low in the sky, Caroline heads to the jutting bluffs near her home and makes her way down the weather-worn steps to the beach below. There's nothing more glorious than watching the sun along "her" stretch of the beach. Palm trees sway in the distance. Sometimes pelicans soar overhead and pause to dip straight down when they spy dinner swimming in the ocean below. Now and then dolphins play in the waves, jumping and diving in formation. This is Caroline's world. So beautiful—sparkling ocean, stately palm trees, sunshine in January, flowers year-round. Surrounded by these good things, she didn't find it hard to believe in God.

Until the cancer hit. Whenever exactly that was. All the time that she had thought she was perfectly fine, it had been spreading destruction inside her. God's beautiful world—a good thing bent out of shape.

WHY? WHY? WHY?

Faced with suffering, fear, and an unknown future, our questions tumble forth.

So what about it, God? Explain yourself. How come I don't see the protection I read about in the Psalms? Where is Your celebrated faithfulness? Where are You, Lord, when I need You most?

Our Christian brothers and sisters see our suffering, and they so want to offer us some ray of hope. So they arm themselves with passages of Holy Scripture to lay on us to prove that we simply *must* be comforted. But we aren't. We know what we feel, and it isn't good. And so we begin to trust our feelings more than we trust biblical truths.

Perhaps you can identify with C. S. Lewis when he wrote in *A Grief Observed*, "Not that I am (I think) in much danger of ceasing to believe in God. The real danger is of coming to believe such dreadful things about Him. The conclusion I dread is not, 'So there's no God after all,' but, 'So this is what God's really like. Deceive yourself no longer.'"[1]

Our fear and pain and human sense of fairness often make us scream, "I don't care about all that pious stuff! I want to be cured right now!"

Philip Yancey in his book *Where Is God When It Hurts?* wrote, "Recently I watched a TV call-in healing program. The biggest applause came when a caller reported his leg was healed just one week before he was scheduled for amputation. The audience shouted, and the emcee declared, 'This is the best miracle we've had tonight!' I couldn't help wondering how many amputees were watching, forlornly wondering where their faith had failed."[2]

Remember Stan, who felt called by God to heal Justin? He made the same point that emcee made. He pointed his finger right in Justin's wife's face and said, "Your problem, Nancy, is that you haven't *insisted* that God make Justin well."

Insisted? To God?

Yes, our questions are understandable. It certainly does sometimes seem as if God allows circumstances into our lives that are harming us, and it does seem that they're without sense or plan. We read the Scripture verses offered us, but they cause us still more confusion: "Ask, and it shall be given you"; "If ye shall ask any thing in my name"; "They shall lay hands on the sick, and they shall recover"; "Who forgiveth all thine iniquities; who healeth all thy diseases."

Anchor me, Lord!

Immovable Anchors

The first thing to do is step back and securely anchor the subject of pain and suffering to an immovable foundation point. Philip Yancey does this well when he writes,

Any discussion of how pain and suffering fit into God's system ultimately leads back to the cross.

By taking it on Himself, Jesus in a sense dignified pain. Of all the kinds of lives He could have lived, He chose a suffering one. Because of Jesus, I can never say about a person, "He must be suffering because of some sin he committed"; Jesus, who did not sin, also felt pain. And I cannot say, "Suffering and death must mean God has forsaken us; He's left us alone to self-destruct." Because even though Jesus died, His death became the great victory of history, pulling man and God together. God made a supreme good out of that awful day.

Jesus' followers are not insulated from the tragedies of this world, just as He was not.[3]

And yet it's quite natural that we try every means available to get our Lord to make everything all right again. To heal us as He healed the sick and dying when He walked on earth. To dry our tears and stop our pain as we know He is so able to do. To patch our lives back together.

Martin Luther once wrote, "Reason holds that if God had a watchful eye on us and loved us, He would prevent all evil and not let us suffer. But now, since all sorts of calamities come to us, we conclude, 'Either God has forgotten me, or God is hostile to me and does not want me.' Against such thoughts, which we harbor by nature, we must arm ourselves with God's Word. We must not judge according to our opinion, but according to the Word."

That's it right there. It is our human logic that trips us up. *If God really, truly cares about me,* we reason, *He won't let anything bad happen to me.*

"Not so fast," God says. He reminds us, "My thoughts are not your thoughts, neither are your ways my ways" (Isa. 55:8-9).

Ask in His Name

"But wait," you may say. "What about John 14:13-14? Those verses are in red letters in my Bible. That means they're words that came right out of Jesus' very own mouth." Here's what they say: "I will do whatever you ask in my name, so that the Son may bring glory to the Father. You may ask me for anything in my name, and I will do it."

Those are great verses, all right. What a promise! But this does not guarantee that God will do anything and everything we ask so long as we add to our prayer the PS: "In Christ's name." No, to pray in Christ's name is to identify with the purpose of Christ to the extent that our will becomes the will of God (1 John 5:14). It may be that the better answer isn't "Yes," but "Yes, if . . ." or "No, although . . ." or sometimes just plain "No."

Working for Good

"What about Rom. 8:28?" you may ask. "'We know that all things work together for good to them that love God, to them who are the called according to his purpose.' [KJV]. What about that? Where's the good in this cancer?"

Ah, look at the verse again. The promise is not that everything that happens to us is good in and of itself. No, it's that *in* everything *God is at work* so that even in our most miserable circumstances, He will produce good.

Rejoice Because . . .

Though you hate the cancer and it causes you great agony, you can rejoice in spite of it. Who but a Christian could say that? Only we who know the extent of this truth: this suffering is far, far from meaningless. Just look at what God is producing in you: "We also rejoice in our sufferings, because we know that suffering produces perseverance; perseverance, character; and character, hope. And hope does not disappoint us, because God has poured out his love into our hearts by the Holy Spirit, whom he has given us" (Rom. 5:3-5).

Mature Wisdom

You have always been an asset to the family of God. I'm sure of that. There are those who have benefited from your example. But, oh, after you have persevered—well, just look at what the apostle James has to say: "Consider it pure joy, my brothers, whenever you face trials of many kinds, because you know that the testing of your faith develops perseverance. Perseverance must finish its work so that you may be mature and complete, not lacking anything" (1:2-4).

More Precious

Take it from one who knew a good bit about suffering: it's not all bad. In Ps. 119:71-72 the psalmist writes, "It was good for me to be afflicted so that I might learn your decrees. The law from your mouth is more precious to me than thousands of pieces of silver and gold."

Now *that's* treasure!

THE HUMAN CONDITION

Here's a foundational truth about suffering: it's a pivotal part of the human condition. One bite of that fruit in the Garden of Eden ruined it for all of us: good, bad, young, old, cute, homely, Christian, pagan. We all suffer, and in the end we all die. Sometimes God chooses to intervene in miraculous ways; sometimes He doesn't.

"I can accept that," Keith confided. "But as a Christian I prayed for healing. I believe I have a right to expect that prayer to be answered."

Belief that there will be a healing can be a great antidote for helplessness. It gives the sufferer not only hope but also a goal. There's also a danger, though. Should God choose not to heal, the person can experience a huge stumbling block to his or her faith. The end result is an even more desperate plunge into helpless despair.

"So what are you saying?" Keith asked. "I shouldn't pray for healing?"

No. Certainly pray. Pray with faith and with hope. But understand that God is under no obligation to answer your prayers on your terms. If you're healed, praise God. If not, understand that God has not let you down. He can use even your infirmity to produce good and wise maturity within you.

"But I'm not just anybody!" you may be saying. "I'm a Christian! I'm a beloved child of God."

I know you are. But consider this: If God were to heal all Christians of their illnesses, it would insulate us and prevent us from identifying with the hurting people of the world. When the apostle Paul begged that his "thorn in the flesh" be removed, God refused. Paul's suffering continued. And what happened as a result? Countless Christians through the ages have a deeper identification with Paul. We feel his pain. When he tells us that God's grace is sufficient, we listen, because we *know* he isn't just spouting platitudes. He's been there.

We know that

- We live in aging bodies. (If you doubt this, compare pictures of yourself over the years. Notice anything?)
- God can use illness for the benefit of the kingdom of God. (We see this demonstrated in a wide range of people from the apostle Paul to Joni Eareckson Tada, the quadriplegic who has had such a profound worldwide ministry.)

Therefore, tread carefully. Don't box God into only one way of responding to your prayers for healing or into having only one "purpose" for your suffering. God is all-knowing. He is wise. He is merciful and loving. And He is God.

As mentioned earlier, there's nothing inherently good about cancer. There's nothing inherently good about famine or war or getting hit by a drunk driver. But God takes all the events of our lives—both the good and the bad—and weaves them together into an intricate pattern of divine perfection. The blessed outcome is good, both for us individually and the general good only God can know.

In *The Problem of Pain*, C. S. Lewis wrote, "We want not so much a father in heaven as a grandfather in heaven—whose plan for the universe was such that it might be said at the end of each day, 'A good time was had by all.'"

Yes, that's pretty much it.

Lewis concludes: "The problem of reconciling human suffering with the existence of God who loves is only insoluble so long as we attach a trivial meaning to the word 'love,' and limit His wisdom by what seems to us to be wise."[4]

ETERNAL ANSWERS

Let's go back to Christ on the Cross.

It was through Jesus Christ that the eternal God of the universe entered humanity. In Jesus, God experienced the world as a man—including its pain and suffering. Humbling himself, He traded in a perfect heavenly body for a frail body of restructured clay, one that was capable of experiencing horrible, torturous, agonizing pain.

Surely the agony of Jesus' crushing humanity peaked when He—the great Teacher of communicating with God, His Heavenly Father, through prayer—realized on the Cross that His own tortured prayers were going unheard. He had already been deserted by men. Now He was deserted by God. *My God, my God,* He cried out in agony we can never begin to comprehend, *why have You forsaken Me?*

Listen to what Caroline says: "I just wish God could visit me personally and give me some answers and explanations. I mean, I want to believe and trust Him. I really do. If I could just see Him once and hear Him state His reasons for putting me through this, I could endure it."

I know how Caroline feels. I've said those very same words more times that I care to remember. But then I think of that statement framed in Christ's agonized words from the Cross. Would it really matter if He were sitting here explaining to me? The real question is "Am I willing to trust Him even when I don't understand? Even when He's not doing it my way? Even when His answer to my plea is "No"?

Ask God to allow you to see from His perspective, for perspective changes everything. Once He enables us to catch a glimpse of eternal perspective, we suddenly realize that fairness through our human eyes is not meant to be balanced. Our perspective focuses on what's transitory, but God's eternal perspective is firmly fixed on what's lasting. Eternal glory, the unveiling of God's master plan—these will last forever. Everything else—numbing pain, tears of fear and exasperation, the ravages of cancer, shouts of "but it isn't fair!"—no matter how earth-shattering it seems today, will be inconsequential in eternity.

So will the scale of justice one day be balanced? Not a chance. It will forever be tremendously skewed in favor of our good and God's glory.

GIVING UP THE DEMANDS

To me, it's a rich spiritual anchor to know I can give up on my demands of God. Holding on to them is too wearing and exhausting an exercise. Instead I want to rest in His arms and claim the riches He has for me. I want to know that when the fire is over, I will emerge refined as silver and pure as gold (Zech. 13:9).

I want to turn my eyes to my Father in heaven and say with the psalmist, "Whom have I in heaven but you? And earth has nothing I desire besides you" (Ps. 73:25).

It just may be that your cancer will be the means of bringing you heart-to-heart close to God. It just may be that this will be a time when you will come to love Him for who He is and not merely for what He'll give you. It just may be that this is the time that will lead you to where you can honestly say, "My flesh and my heart fail, but God is the strength of my heart and my portion forever" (v. 26).

Confess your doubts and fears to God, and let go of them. Then move forward through faith in the One who gave His life for you. Keep your eyes firmly fixed upon the One who works all things together for your good and His glory.

Unless the Lord returns first, my body is one day going to give way to physical death. The same is true for you. Whether the length of our days is short or long, not one of us will be short-changed by God. He's cheating no one. Facing our own mortality helps bring into focus the reality of eternal life through Jesus Christ.

The apostle Paul understood this when he wrote, "Our citizenship is in heaven, from which also we eagerly wait for a Savior, the Lord Jesus Christ; who will transform the body of our humble state into conformity with the body of His glory, by the exertion of the power that He has even to subject all things to Himself" (Phil. 3:20-21, NASB).

Know it. Expect it. Look forward to it. That doesn't mean to give up on this life. No, this is where God has you today. But it does mean to "set your mind on things above, not on earthly things" (Col. 3:2).

Nick was devastated by his diagnosis of esophageal cancer. "I'm only 46!" he said. "I'm in the prime of my life! Just when I'm starting to reap the benefits of so many years of struggle and work—well, it just isn't fair!"

Then one day, as Nick sat in the cancer center waiting for his chemo treatment, he struck up a conversation with Robert.

"That young man was so angry," Nick recalled of the 23-year-old student. "Yet I was really drawn to him. I mean, why shouldn't he be bitter? All his studying, all his preparation, and now his life was pulled up short."

Enter Holly, a skinny, bald six-year-old skipping over to the water fountain for a drink. She had her worn-out stuffed kitty firmly clutched in her little hand. Both Nick and Robert fell silent as Holly flashed them a big smile, sans front teeth.

"At least I had my childhood," Robert said quietly.

Why you? Why *not* you?

Why now? Well, why not *before* now?

None of us can expect to live an entire lifetime free of disappointment and suffering. None of us can hope to escape loss and pain. We expect to live in a society in which good is rewarded and bad is punished. When this doesn't happen, we cry out, "But it isn't fair!"

I for one wouldn't want to live in a perfectly fair world. There wouldn't be any grace in such a world, for grace is grace only when it's undeserved.

Please, God, spare me a life of graceless fairness! It terrifies me to contemplate what it would be like to always get just what I deserve. How infinitely better to live in a world with unmerited favor!

That's the world Paul was referring to when he wrote, "I pray that you . . . may . . . grasp . . . how wide and long and high and deep is the love of Christ" (Eph. 3:17-18).

That, my friend, is the world of grace.

10

WILL I EVER BE WHOLE AGAIN?

Jen's journey through chemotherapy and on to a subsequent bone marrow transplant was more horrendously arduous than she could ever have imagined. But she survived. There has been no sign of her cancer for over four years. Two years ago she gave birth to a second daughter, Kaylee Ann. To see Jen riding her bike around town with her two-year old in tow, or watching her play on a soccer team with now-teenager LeeAnn or roughhousing with nine-year-old Ryan, you would never guess that just four years ago she was in a desperate fight for her life.

"It's over!" LeeAnn says happily of her mom's battle with cancer.

Jen knows better. When the kids are all out of earshot Jen says, "It's never really over. It's like the sword of Damocles hanging over my head for the rest of my life."

Not everyone is as candid as Jen. Yet to one degree or another, few cancer survivors can honestly say they're able to look at the future without the fear of relapse.

"I finished my treatments and just assumed it was over," Myra said. "I never thought about having a recurrence. No one in the cancer center ever talked about that. Then my friend Sherry, who had a stem cell transplant and had boosted me through all my treatments, Sherry, who had walked beside me and cried with me and prayed with me and talked and listened endlessly on the phone, Sherry had a recurrence. I couldn't believe it!"

Myra's Bible study leader was the one who broke the

news to her. "Sherry has cancer again, Myra," she said, "and it doesn't look good."

Myra was shocked into silence. She, too, could get it again!

The next day, Myra went to Sherry's house to see her. Sherry was terribly distressed. "I'm not going to be a grandmother," she said mournfully, even though her sons weren't even married yet.

"She had been my rock of Gibraltar," Myra said. "It was she who had walked me through everything. Her hair fell out, then came back curly, and so did mine. She was positive she was cured, and so was I. But now Sherry was going to die. What was I going to do?"

Then there was Marguerite. She and Myra got to know each other while they sat together in the chemotherapy department waiting for their chemo treatments. Over time, they worked through so many difficult things together. It had been a while since the two had seen each other, so Myra was excited to run into Marguerite in a coffee shop.

"Marguerite looked wonderful, all dressed up in a suit and ready to take on the world," recalled Myra. "She was wondering if she should go to Europe with her son, and I said, 'Yes, yes, yes!' I was so excited for her. Then she said, 'The doctors think I should because it might be my last chance.' Two months later, Marguerite died."

And there was Jesse, who sat with Myra through radiation every single day of her treatment. "He was my first friend in the radiation department, and I talked to him so much about the Lord," Myra recalled. "One weekend, half way through our radiation treatment, he got married. He was so excited and happy!"

But Jesse died also.

"All of a sudden, all these people who were so much a part of me were dying," Myra said, shaking her head.

From then on, when it was time for a checkup, Myra would get on the Internet and begin obsessively researching colon cancer. "Oh, no," she would fret. "It's going to come back! I know this time the doctor will find something, and it'll be back!" She would become more and more frantic until she was totally overcome by panic. Then, barely holding together, she would go in for the appointment—and there was no cancer. She would breathe a sigh of relief and struggle to get herself back together. But it was only a matter of time before the entire cycle started over again.

Finally one day, Myra looked at her doctor and said, "I can't live my life like this any more. I've decided I'm just going to be recovered and in remission, and that's it. No more ups and downs with every appointment.

"Absolutely, Myra," the doctor replied. "How else can you live life but to just think it isn't going to come back? And then if it does, we'll deal with it. But in the meantime, you will just assume it won't."

Myra no longer takes someone along to her doctor's appointments because she no longer needs the moral support. In fact, she's developed a helpful routine: "I stop at my favorite Mexican restaurant and have lunch. Then I go up to the doctor's office, and he tells me I'm fine. I'm careful not to yell and scream on the way out, because I don't want to scare the sick people, but once outside I call Tim on the cell phone and shriek out, 'I made it! I made it again!' Then I hang up and go home."

"Hey, wait!" you may be saying. "Myra can't just determine that she's going to be fine. There's no assurance it will work out like that."

No, there certainly isn't. But, hey—life really doesn't hold any assurances on the physical level for any of us on anything, does it?

"I refuse to compromise my life with worry," Marlene insisted. "Someday I'll die of something, but I can assure you it won't be of worry. Whether I have 30 days or 30 years, I will live my life to the fullest." And she does. It's been 22 years since she was first diagnosed with breast cancer.

DO NOT WORRY

Jesus had some interesting comments about worry. In Matt. 6:27 He asked, *Who of you by worrying can add a single hour to his life?* Evidently not a single one of his listeners raised a hand, because in verse 34 He said, "Therefore do not worry about tomorrow, for tomorrow will worry about itself. Each day has enough trouble of its own."

That's for sure! I for one don't need any more worries today!

BUT DO BE WISE

Jesus was certainly not advocating that we be foolhardy in how we handle today. Yes, the risk of a recurrence of your cancer does exist. And it's possible that another type of cancer might develop. Therefore, it's vital that you be scrupulous about your follow-up care. This means

- Follow doctors' orders!
- Pay attention to and follow up on your physical checkups.
- Ask what activites are good for you; then do them regularly.
- Ask if there are things you can do to reduce the chances of a recurrence.
- Stay as far away from toxic people as you possibly can.

If you give yourself permission to quit the constant worrying about something, after a while you won't think about it every single day. In time, you'll be able to get through a long time without thinking about it at all. But you can never forget it completely. To paraphrase a famous saying about freedom, the price of health is eternal vigilance.

"No one ever pretended there was a chance. I wondered myself," said Theo. "Lung cancer is a notoriously deadly disease. I didn't give up worrying as I recited Ps. 31:15— 'My times are in your hands.' But I didn't give up constantly searching for new advances, either. And it paid off."

Theo learned of a cancer-screening device developed at

the University of Maryland School of Medicine that could help detect the recurrence of lung cancer.

"It's a win-win situation," Theo says. "It increases my chances of survival, and it gives me a chance to help others who will suffer from this disease."

Keep Your Body in Fighting Shape

Too often cancer survivors end up no better informed about the importance of diet, exercise, and other factors that can affect their health than they were before they got sick. The emphasis has been on getting rid of the cancer, and too often it stops there. Determine that you won't settle for "just as good as before." Why not "better than ever"? Keep your body healthy and your immune system strong by committing yourself to doing the following:

- Eat well. But don't make your diet yet another source of stress. Don't feel obligated to eat foods you dislike or guilty about eating foods you dearly love. You need to enjoy life!
- Keep yourself well hydrated. Make it a hard-and-fast rule to drink at least six to eight glasses of spring water a day. The difficult part isn't drinking it—it's getting into the habit.
- Get regular exercise. Settle on something you enjoy so that it's pleasant—if not downright fun—rather than a duty.
- Avoid too much physical stress. Set boundaries and insist that other people respect then. Learn to say no. (I'm still struggling with this one.)
- Reduce emotional stress. Stress takes a terrible toll on your body's well-being. In chapter 11 we'll talk more about ways to reduce stress.
- Watch your weight. Don't diet; just eat smart.
- Keep a positive attitude. You can do this. When you do, you'll find it well worth the effort.
- Make prayer a regular and enjoyable part of your life.

Would you like to get a jump-start on getting into

shape? Here's a suggestion: Do it right now. Today. Try this immediacy out on Col. 3:12-25. Read this passage including the word *today* with each verse:

- "Let the peace of Christ rule in your hearts" *today* (v. 15).
- "Let the word of Christ dwell in you richly" *today* (v. 16).

Along with the specific instructions given to wives, husbands, children, and fathers (vv. 18-21), include the word *today* with each one.

"One thing about cancer," said Marlene, "is that for these past 22 years it's caused me to live each day as though it were my last—not to worry and fret about it, but to appreciate and enjoy it as though I wouldn't get the chance again."

Live Today

"Peace I leave with you; my peace I give you," Jesus said in John 14:27. "I do not give to you as the world gives. Do not let your hearts be troubled and do not be afraid."

Peace—what a concept!

Later He said, "I have told you these things, so that in me you may have peace. In this world you will have trouble. But take heart! I have overcome the world" (John 16:33).

Let me suggest something that may go against everything your industrious parents and your keep-your-eyes-on-eternity Sunday School teachers ever taught you: Live for today. No, I don't mean to be selfish or self-centered or grabby or to clean out your family's checking account. I just mean to enjoy yourself and your loved ones today so you don't end up joining the ranks of those who forever sacrifice for a future that never seems to get here. Marguerite finally made it back to her family home in Europe, but just barely, and only because her doctor ordered, "Just go! Now!"

When you do those things, you'll find it much easier to put away the killer "what ifs":

- What if I don't live to wear that second pair of running shoes in my closet?
- What if I'm not well enough to attend the reunion I've already paid for?
- What if I never live to see my grandchildren?
- What if I never even get married?

"I'm no example," Justin says. "Goodness knows how I've struggled with this and how I'm still struggling. But I think I can honestly say my greatest health problem today is not cancer. It's the aches and pains of arthritis!"

11
REST AND DE-STRESS

"The worst of my treatment was over," recalled Myra. "Now I was just exhausted. More than anything, I wanted rest and cooperation from my family. But everything I said and did seemed to irritate my oldest son. *I* seemed to irritate him. Whatever I'd say, he'd say something back, and we'd be in an argument. In the past, I had always been his chauffeur. Now that I was grounded, so was he. One afternoon he came out to the patio where I was lying on a chaise lounge in the sunshine. Without so much as a how-are-you-feeling-Mom? he informed me, 'I need you to take me to Hendrey's Beach.' I told him he was quite aware that I couldn't drive. He angrily retorted, 'You never take me anywhere!' then stormed off."

When the apostle Paul wrote to the church at Philippi, "Be anxious for nothing" (4:6, NKJV), it's obvious he didn't have a teenage son! But then, he was in a Roman prison, and *that* would certainly cause a good bit of anxiety!

Let's face it: life is stressful—with or without teenagers, with or without Roman soldiers out to get your head, with or without cancer. It's impossible to live a totally stress-free life unless you completely close yourself off. Actually, some people try to do exactly that, but even they seem eventually to find things to get stressed about.

When you're stressed, your body reacts as though it's being physically threatened. It immediately releases hormones that restrict the flow of blood to your body tissues. This diminished blood flow means less oxygen and a greater buildup of carbon dioxide, which sets up a fertile ground for cancer cells to grow and prosper. So the more

nonstop stress you endure and the more fever pitch its level, the greater the damage done to your immune system.

"But there are a lot of stressors in my life that I just
can't do anything about," you may say.

True. You can't kick a selfish kid out of the house. You
can't reason with the Roman Empire. You can't quit your
job if you need the money or the insurance it provides. You
can't dump a family member who's giving you grief. You
certainly can't do anything about terrorist bombings or
earthquakes or famine or pestilence or war. For those unal-
terable stressors you can look to Reinhold Neibuhr's "Serenity Prayer," which asks for the "serenity to accept the
things I cannot change; courage to change the things I can;
and wisdom to know the difference."

There are, however, many stressors over which you do
have some control, and it's here you need to take action.
Perhaps you should change jobs. Maybe there are some
people—even family members—from whom you would
do well to separate yourself. Maybe it would be a good
idea to turn off the evening news and drop your news
magazine subscription for a while.

Maybe you can even refuse to stress over what other
people think about what you say or do or how you look.
To this day, Myra changes her hairstyle so often people are
always exclaiming, "Myra, every time I see you, you look
different!" She breezily responds, "I know. I'm always rein-
venting myself." If she feels like a redhead, she's a redhead. Tomorrow she may be a blond. "Who really cares?"
she says. "Not me. I know what it's like to have no hair.
Sort of puts the hair thing in perspective, doesn't it?"

PEACE IN PLACE OF ANXIETY

On many a dark, lonely night everything seemed out of
control to David, who had never been anything but a humble shepherd boy. The prophet Samuel had anointed him
king of Israel, yet he was forever on the run from the mur-

derous King Saul, hiding in caves, fearing for his life. Doubts assailed him. Fears smothered him. There seemed to him to be no escape. Night after night he tossed and turned just as we do. Like us, he railed at the seeming unfairness of suffering. But in his doubts and fears, his mind blurred with questions, he turned to his great Shepherd and reminded himself of the Lord's presence. Recalling what he already knew to be true brought peace to his troubled soul.

Come peek over David's shoulder and read some of what he wrote:

> The LORD is my Shepherd, I shall not be in want.
>> He makes me lie down in green pastures,
> he leads me beside quiet waters,
>> he restores my soul.
> He guides me in paths of unrighteousness
>> for his name's sake.
> Even though I walk
>> through the valley of the shadow of death,
> I will fear no evil,
>> for you are with me;
> your rod and your staff,
>> they comfort me.
> You prepare a table before me
>> in the presence of my enemies.
> You anoint my head with oil;
>> my cup overflows.
> Surely goodness and love will follow me
>> all the days of my life,
> and I will dwell in the house of the LORD
>> forever *(Ps. 23:1-6).*

David knew. "Because He is at my right hand," he wrote in Ps. 16:8, "I shall not be moved."

You may not have the silver pen of David the psalmist, but you can still talk to God. You can talk to Him about your concerns for yourself and your family, about your conflicts and challenges, about your frustrations.

Worry can do a lot of things *to* you: Prayer can do a lot of things *for* you.

Work toward consciously replacing the stressors in your life with positives. Fill your life with the things that will help you do that:

- **True Security.** There's only one source of real security, and that's the unconditional love found in a personal relationship with Jesus Christ. It's here that a life free of anxiety begins.
- **Forgiveness.** You'll be amazed at how much stress evaporates when you give up the grudges from the past. Let go of old frustrations and anger. This is not only physically healthful but also scripturally sound. God forgives us our sins and cleanses us from all unrighteousness. He also commands us to forgive others.
- **Acceptance of what is.** You can't change what is. But you can change yourself and your attitude toward the new givens in your life.
- **Responsibility.** You can relax and de-stress, even if you're a type-A personality. These are choices you make. You can't count on others to make them for you, and you don't have the right to blame them if they don't. Take responsibility for giving good care to yourself.
- **Draw Close to the Lord.** Make it a top priority to draw close to Him. Spend time praying and reading God's Word. Become involved in the fellowship of your local body of believers and in a small, supportive Bible study group.

QUICK FIXES

It never hurts to pad your stress-free, positive life with some quick-fix "play time" ideas. Here are some of my personal favorites:

- Play a game you loved as a child. (Checkers and jacks are my picks.)

- Color in a coloring book.
- Buy a bird feeder, and keep a log of all the birds you see.
- Take a warm bubble bath. (If you don't like baths, do something else luxuriously lazy.)
- Stay up past your usual bedtime and do some stargazing.
- Chew bubble gum and blow bubbles.

You may not care for my ideas. That's fine. Make your own list. The thing is to plan ahead and be prepared with some quick relaxers.

RELAX DEEPLY

Sometimes the best thing you can do for yourself is to let your mind and body restore and heal through deep relaxation. Watching television doesn't count. Neither does reading books or magazines or talking with someone. All these activities require your mind to remain active. In order to relax deeply, you must consciously enter a state in which both your body and your mind become quiet and tranquil. Only then can the restoration begin.

STRESS MANAGEMENT DOS

You say you're no stress management expert? Join the crowd. Still, here are seven "dos" that will get you headed in the right direction:

1. Learn to say no. You can say it kindly. You can say it with a smile on your face. You can say it in Christian love. Just say it!
2. Practice relaxation skills. Take slow, deep breaths. Say calming, soothing things to yourself. Consciously relax your body from the top of your head to the tips of your toes.
3. Listen to soothing music.
4. Read nurturing, uplifting books and articles.
5. Pray contemplatively, and meditate on scripture. Ps.

119:165 promises, *Great peace have they who love your law.*

6. Practice flexibility. Life will not always go as you plan. Expect it, and don't be thrown.
7. Laugh lots at lots of different things—sometimes even at yourself.

When Jen was in isolation awaiting a bone marrow transplant, her husband saw how miserable she was and determined to cheer her up. He started a laugh file for her, cutting out comic strips and humorous columns he thought she would especially enjoy. He even copied down bloopers from anywhere he found them, including, for example, their minister's accidental Sunday morning greeting: "Welcome to this morning's circus" (service).

Friends and family soon caught the bug, and Jen's laugh file grew and grew. "Whenever I was down, I could open up that file and read all those funny, silly things again and count on a good hour's worth of laughter," Jen said, a smile spreading across her face from just remembering it. "It did me more good than a whole pharmacy full of medicine!"

Rest

Sometimes the best antidote for anxiety is simply to rest. We grow weary physically, emotionally, and spiritually. And in each area we need to rest.

Physical rest. This one seems easy enough—just lie down and take a nap! Yes, physical rest does include time for sleep and leisure, but it's more than just that. It also involves good nutrition, regular exercise, and relaxation. It means knowing when to say, "That's enough work" and calling it a day.

Emotional rest. Ah, emotional rest. This is the peace, quiet, contentment, and refreshment of spirit we've been talking about, as opposed to anxiety, stress, and fear.

Spiritual rest. It's strange that this type of rest tends to be so neglected when we all long for it in the deepest part of our beings. It's here we finally get rest from our guilt, doubt, confusion, and despair. We long for the peace of God that transcends all understanding that the apostle Paul talks about in Phil. 4:7. We achieve it by obeying the instruction to cast all our cares upon our Father God because He cares for us (1 Pet. 5:7).

To-Do List

Let's end this chapter by developing a personal semi-official rest-and-anti-stress to-do list.

Begin by listing the 10 most important priorities for the rest of your life.

Here's the first half of my list:

1. Play with my grandchildren while they still want to play with me.
2. Memorize passages of Scripture that move me to tears, such as Rom. 8 and Isa. 53.
3. Travel to places that increase my understanding of and appreciation for people in other cultures. Allow those people and places to affect the way I live my life.
4. Walk on the beach regularly, not for exercise, but because it restores my soul.
5. Read books on all kinds of subjects that stretch my mind, move me emotionally, and stir my curiosity.

When you have all 10 things listed, go back and relist the items in the order of their importance.

This was hard, but I reordered my half-list this way:

1. Play with my grandchildren while they still want to play with me. (I figured this should be number 1 since it has such a limited window of opportunity. The oldest is already 9! She loves to have me around now, but in three or four years . . .)
2. Travel to places that increase my understanding of and appreciation for people in other cultures. Allow those people and places to affect the way I live my life. (I must do this now! This kind of travel isn't like

taking a cruise ship. It's rough. I may not be able to do it in 10 years, 5 years, or maybe even next year.)

3. Memorize passages of Scripture that move me to tears, such as Rom. 8 and Isa. 53. (The sooner the better! My memory isn't getting any sharper!)

4. Read books on all kinds of subjects that stretch my mind, move me emotionally, and stir my curiosity. (This will help me be successful in other areas of my life.)

5. Walk on the beach regularly, not for exercise, but because it restores my soul. (This is the easiest to accomplish and the thing that comes the most naturally, so I don't think it needs a high priority.)

Finished? Now go back and assign each item a stress level from 1 (almost no stress at all) to 10 (soaring stress).

Then also give each item a value level from 1 (lowest) to 10 (highest). Here's mine:

	Stress Level	Value Level
1. Playing with grandkids	4	9
2. Travel	9	9
3. Memorizing scripture	5	8
4. Reading	2	6
5. Walk on the beach	3	7

Now balance the stress level of a particular item with its value level.

On items in which the stress is low and value high (such as reading and walking on the beach), the go-ahead is clear and inviting. Even those that fall in the middle aren't difficult. But what about when the stress is high?

On Caroline's list, her top priority was to see her daughter married. The stress level of planning a wedding was extremely high—Caroline assigned it a 9. But the value? It earned a full 10. Even though the stress was high, the value was even higher. The wedding was well worth the stress.

The second highest item on my list, traveling, is the same way. Next month I leave for China, India, and Indonesia, where I will be interviewing women who are actively persecuted for their faith in Christ. Stressful? You bet! But I can't think of anything I would rather be doing—except perhaps playing with the grandchildren.

"I'm a businessman," said Justin. "I always have been, and I guess I always will be. Making the most of my tax advantages has always been stressful, so I assigned it a 9 on my stress list. But I also gave it an 8 on my value list."

That could be a hard item to reconcile. But Justin found a way.

"This year I found a way to make the value of my tax decisions far outweigh the stress that went into it. I decided to invest in the education of each of the third-generation children of our family. There are eight children between the ages of six months and 15 years who are going to have Christmas presents of tax-free college scholarships in their stockings. Stress-free tax preparation for me? Hardly. But what a value for my buck! The future of my extended family, my strong commitment to education, the wisdom of planning, well—I got it all. Every night I think about it as I get ready for bed and I go to sleep with a grin on my face."

De-stress doesn't mean the absence of stress. It means the ability to handle the stress wisely.

12
A Place to Grow

"From the morning I woke up unable to open my left eye or speak a coherent sentence, I thought of little but getting through this and coming out alive," Justin said. "I'd never thought about 'afterward.' I was far too wound up in the 'here and now.'"

But now Justin is a survivor. And so are you. Now that you have joined the community of brokenness and survival, you have earned the right both to speak and to be heard. It may not be a position you would have sought out, but because of what you have been through, you're in a perfect place to help relieve the suffering around you by comforting others and offering them hope. People around you will be drawn near to the kingdom of God by watching God at work in your life.

"I love to go out and help other people who are struggling with the things I struggle with," Myra says. "I have so much compassion for where they are. I long to talk to them, to be their friend, to give them the hope of Christ."

The interesting thing is, Myra is a multifaceted person with all kinds of experiences that give her common ground with a wide variety of people. For instance, she has adopted children, so she could certainly go out and share wholeheartedly with others who have adopted or who are adopting. But for some reason she just doesn't have the same vitality for those folks as she has for ones who are battling cancer.

"The cancer just drives you to your knees," Myra says. "You have no way in your own strength to fix it. If you can't conceive a child, it's a terrible disappointment, but you can find a way to fix it. You can take it into your own hands, and you can make something happen. With cancer, you can't. You're so helpless it knocks you right down onto your knees."

Because of her firm stand on abortion, Myra had long been known in her community as being staunchly right wing. She ran for a position on the school board and took strong positions against such things as outcome-based education. Everywhere her name was used, it was stamped "conservative." One woman in town we'll call Jane was an outspoken school board rival of Myra's and bitterly opposed to everything she stood for. She detested Myra's conservative views and took every opportunity to hold her up to ridicule. Whenever Myra would make a presentation, Jane would be sure to attend and seat herself in a prominent place. Then she would ask questions intended to incite and inflame emotions against Myra and her positions.

Myra and Jane's paths had not crossed for years, yet the year after Myra's bout with cancer, she ran into Jane at a Christmas party.

"You probably don't remember me," Jane said to Myra.

"Oh, yes I do, Jane," Myra said. "How have you been?" And the two began a casual chat.

"So what are you doing now?" Jane asked.

"Well," Myra said, "I spent the last year or so battling cancer. Actually, I'm just getting back on my feet."

Immediately Jane's demeanor changed. Suddenly she was filled with compassion and concern.

Myra explains: "Cancer takes away all that stupid stuff in our lives that makes us not like people. We can have heart-to-heart conversations we never could have had before."

A CITY SET ON A HILL

Now that you're set high on the hill of experience, your witness cannot be hidden. Cancer gives you a unique authority to "preach the Word; be prepared in season and out of season; correct, rebuke and encourage—with great patience and careful instruction" (2 Tim. 4:2). Will you always feel like it? No! Sometimes you'll feel downright downcast and depressed. But it just may be that God will use those "out of season" moments even more powerfully than He uses what you consider to be the "in season" ones.

Emily is a city set on a hill. Just 32 when she began an extraordinarily aggressive treatment for breast cancer, she was overwhelmed by the side effects.

"I just wanted to live for my children," she said. "They were so little." When doctors told her they had done all they could for her, Emily was devastated. She had never believed in alternative therapies, but now she pulled out all the stops. Most important, she prayed. She prayed and she prayed and she prayed. This past year she celebrated a day doctors said she would never live to see—her 42nd birthday.

"Why am I still alive?" Emily asks. "Because God isn't done with me yet. Maybe He wants me to use my experiences as a patient to help others."

She certainly is doing just that.

"I can offer more than just information," she says earnestly. "I can offer hope."

Hope. Love. A sense of presence. These are the resources you have to offer suffering people.

And who on earth understands how to offer them? The person who has experienced it and has come through wrapped in the blanket of God's comfort. You have endured the painful experience, and you're the very best counselor God can use.

Those who are coming along the cancer journey behind you need what you have to offer. They need to talk about the possibility of dying. Most people will avoid the subject. They want to be hopeful, of course, and they don't want to upset the person who's already hurting. But you know what those others don't know: the fact that talking about dying, especially to someone who knows the Lord, is actually a really helpful activity.

Those who are coming along behind you also want to talk about all the things they're really sad about. For instance, Myra talked with Elena, a young mother of five who was really upset about the prospects of not seeing her children marry and give her grandchildren. She couldn't think of anything else. Myra told her, "Nothing can take that away from you, Elena. You are your children's mother, so whenever they have children, you'll be their grandmother. Even if you're no longer on this earth, you will still be their grandmother."

Elena was really into crafts and said, "But I so wish I could make some things for them."

"Well, why not do it now and leave it for them?" Myra suggested. And that's just what Elena has done. Her husband made her a cedar chest, and she set it up for her future grandchildren. In it are several special handmade outfits from her homeland of Guatemala and two dark-haired dolls. She is now halfway through a quilt she is making with traditional Guatemalan designs.

Justin said, "When my treatments ended and I had passed my two-year survival checkup, the cancer center contacted me. They asked if I was willing to be in their buddy program. Most new cancer patients are terrified and confused, their brains reeling with the enormity of the diagnosis. So the center likes to buddy-up new patients with old-hand volunteers who can calm down the new guys and walk them through the procedure. I asked straight out, 'Am I free to talk about the Lord?' And they said, 'Yes, absolutely.'"

Justin has been called several times, and he says he's always straightforward about his faith. "I tell them that this is the time to look at what's really important. Then I ask, 'Do you have a relationship with God? Do you know God? Will you tell me about it?' Most people are totally willing. If they're not, I don't push it."

"I'm completely willing to talk to others," said Nick, "and I do get called. There seems to be a lot of esophageal cancer out there." He finds it especially difficult to talk with young men, however. "I just feel so consumed with the 'Why? Why? Why?' questions I wrestled with myself." He understands it's not our call, but it's a very emotional thing to Nick. "It's not rational, and you may think it's not very spiritual, but I've had to ask them to call me just for older guys. I'm great with them, but I can't do the younger ones."

No one has to be all things to all people.

Because she's single, Caroline knows what it's like to go through cancer treatments alone. She's especially good at working with people who have no one close to them.

You may be protesting, "But I'm not a preacher!"

That's fine. When you speak of Jesus Christ, it need not be in a preachy way. Just talk about Him as you would talk about any other dear and beloved friend.

JOIN A SUPPORT GROUP

A support group can be helpful both for what you have to offer and what you will receive. Ultimately, no one else—not family members, nor friends, nor physicians—can know how the cancer journey feels. Don't underestimate the importance of making contact with people who have first-hand knowledge of what it's like to actually walk that journey. You would have much to share with one another. In a support group you'll find an extraordinary opportunity both to give and receive advice, wisdom, and caring support.

"Everyone told me, 'Well, that's behind you now,'" Emily said. "They seem to think the cancer was just an inconvenient interlude in my life and that now I should just pick up and carry on as if nothing happened. Well, that's not all that easy to do."

Of course not. But with the intensity of the onset and frantic treatment schedule behind you, it's easy to feel pushed into getting back to normal.

In Keith's family, it was his wife, Linda, who first went to a support group—one for spouses. It wasn't until a year later, with the couple on the verge of bankruptcy and headed toward a divorce, that Keith finally agreed to go to a group for cancer sufferers.

"I had no idea I was carrying so much anger and resentment," Keith said. "I'm seeing a counselor now and I'm still in a support group. I'm learning to accept myself and my disease, and I'm reaching out a bit to others. The random acts of kindness from strangers have been heartwarming."

Despite the obvious courage of cancer patients, some people feel a real sense of shame about their disease. Some are plagued by guilt for having survived while others didn't. It's in a support group that you can talk about these feelings with others who say, "You too? I feel that way too!"

Certainly not every support group is a good one. Here are some guidelines to help you decide whether a group is right for you:

- Be sure that it does not discourage the use of conventional medical treatment.
- If you're still in cancer treatment yourself, discuss your participation with your doctor or another doctor who's familiar with the work of the group.
- Quickly leave any group that blames participants for their cancer.
- Quickly leave any group in which everyone is gloomy and depressed.
- A Christian support group—one that adheres to biblical principles—is ideal. But this is not always available. At the very least, choose one that does not diminish, negate, or ridicule your biblical beliefs.

To find a support group, call the Wellness Community nearest you or the national organization in Santa Monica, California (310-314-2555), or Make Today Count (800-432-2273) or Cancer Care (212-221-3300). You may also contact the American Cancer Society or the National Cancer Institute. (See the Appendix for contact information.)

PRACTICE THANKFULNESS

When you're sick and depressed and concerned for your life, thankfulness is not an easy attitude to develop. We like to be comfortable. And so we easily interpret as punishment from God harshness of any kind of tough circumstances. We see clear skies and warm sunshine, good health and pleasant living, as signs of God's favor and therefore reasons for thanksgiving. But what about challenges? What about discomfort? What about things that are downright nasty?

"For the first part of my cancer treatments I was not a thankful person," Jen admitted. "I grumbled and I whined and I complained. I was miserable and I made sure everyone else was miserable too. One day when I was in isolation—when I was at my very lowest and most miserable—I couldn't stop crying. I sobbed and sobbed until I cried myself to sleep. When I woke up, my bed had been freshened and a pot of pink geraniums placed on my nightstand. *Thank You, God, that I have a clean bed to lie in,* I whispered in spite of myself. I could see rain beating against the window. *And thank You that I'm warm and dry. And thank You for these beautiful pink geraniums.* From that day on I started and ended each day thanking God for something. I was afraid I might run out of things to say 'Thank You' for, but I never did."

You are a city set on a hill that cannot be hidden.

You, dear friend, can choose to be a channel of God's love, joy, peace, and comfort to the hurting. And you will be blessed for it.

13

LIVING A REFOCUSED LIFE

Santa Barbara, California, is a gathering place for all kinds of people, including the well-known. It isn't unusual to glance up from your morning coffee and see someone at the next table you saw the night before on your video screen, or to find yourself standing at a store cash register behind a music legend. One man in particular who frequents the steep Santa Barbara hills, never touched by winter snows, is cyclist Lance Armstrong.

Back in 1996, Armstrong, then the current top-rated competitive cyclist, announced that his previously diagnosed testicular cancer had spread to his lungs and brain. Doctors put his chances of survival at less than 50 percent. He immediately underwent the most aggressive form of chemotherapy available, an exhausting treatment regimen that left him physically weakened. Yet five months later he was back in training.

Armstrong did not see his ordeal as a death knell. Not at all. Instead, he saw it as a personalized wake-up call. Determined that his brush with death would be turned into something positive, he started the Lance Armstrong Foundation, a nonprofit organization that provides funds for cancer research, awareness, and early detection. And he was back on his bike.

Armstrong had already won the greatest cycling race of all, the Tour de France. Now, after fighting for his life, he went back for another try at the grueling race. Courage? Yes! Indomitable spirit? Yes! Determination to win? Absolutely—but not at all costs. In the 13th stage of the Tour de France, Armstrong's chief rival somersaulted into a creek. Instead of grabbing the chance to zip on past, Armstrong slowed and waited for him to get back onto the road. Then, when the playing field was again level, he proceeded to take over the race in his own right. For the second time, Lance Armstrong won the bicyclist's race of races.

THE REST OF YOUR LIFE

So what are you going to do with the rest of your life? Returning to your regular world after surviving cancer, it has been said, is much like reentering the earth's atmosphere from space. It takes a period of adjustment. And forever after, because of your journey, your eyes are opened to things most people never comprehend. Your perspective has been changed forever.

"I never had a so-called 'life verse,'" says Theo, "but I do now. It's Isaiah 33:2—'O LORD, be gracious to us; we long for you. Be our strength every morning, our salvation in time of distress.'"

A wonderful thing about surviving is that you reach the point at which you begin to search for a new life, one that depends less on circumstances and more on the depths of eternal reality. And, oh, what a doorway to possibility and perspective and ideas that will be!

"My brother Edwin insists I had a crisis of identity," says Theo.

Edwin is probably right. And such an identity crisis may well lead to the formation of a new identity that embraces the loss right into it. The thing is, loss creates a new set of circumstances in which we now must live. When in time we're able to acknowledge the true nature of those circumstances, we can finally begin to forge a new life for ourselves. That's the blessed reality of survival.

Denise, a competitive skier who had a passion for beach volleyball, lost her left leg to cancer. During a time of feeling especially sorry for herself, she ended up pouring out her story to a stranger in a coffee shop. Instead of the gasps of shocked sympathy Denise had expected, the woman asked matter-of-factly, "So how old were you when you got cancer?"

"Thirty-six," Denise said with a sigh. "And you should have seen me before. Skiing, volleyball, running, surfing— I was always on the go."

"Wow—36 years of fun!" the woman said. Then she asked, "Do you have a family?"

"Oh, yes," Denise said. "My husband has been so wonderfully supportive. And my children too. They're teenagers now, really great kids. I couldn't ask for a better family."

After a few moments of silence, the woman looked at Denise and said, "You've had a much fuller life than most of us ever have. I'm so happy for you. Please say a prayer for me." Then, with tears brimming in her eyes, she jumped up and was gone.

"I wish I could say that slap of reality would last me the rest of my life," Denise says, "but I'm a pretty slow learner. I'm afraid I'll have to be reminded now and again just how blessed I really am."

"The rest of my life is going to be way different!" said Marlene. "Before cancer, I didn't just cry over spilled milk —I yelled and screamed over it! I didn't just sweat the small stuff—I perspired over *everything*! I hovered over the children to see if they loaded the dishwasher correctly. I got annoyed if my husband didn't do a job fast enough. I irritably counted the items in the basket of the shopper ahead of me in the express line, and if there was even one too many, I mumbled complaints under my breath."

Cancer changed all that. Today Marlene lives life one day at a time at a more mellow pace. "And there has been a wonderful side benefit," Marlene adds. "My family has followed my lead. We've become a kinder, gentler family."

This Far by Faith

Years ago I read a short story fictitiously set during the life of Lazarus after he had been raised from the dead by Jesus. According to the story, nothing, not even the horrific persecution the Christian Church was suffering, could remove the peaceful smile from Lazarus's face. Finally the furious emperor personally had Lazarus gagged and tied to a wooden stake with kindling piled at its base. As a lighted torch was touched to the tender dry twigs, the emperor ordered, "Take off his gag! I want to see what happens to that smile when he feels those flames."

The gag was removed and the fire lit. As the flames engulfed Lazarus, he laughed out loud and cried out, "Praise God! Oh, praise God!"

What caused this response that so unnerved the Roman emperor? Lazarus had seen eternity! Why should he be afraid? He knew exactly where he was headed, and he was ready to go.

The fact of the matter is, everyone is dying, and everyone needs a Savior. The Bible reveals Jesus Christ alone as worthy of your trust. We'll all die some day if He doesn't come back first. Death is inevitable. God gave us amazingly remarkable bodies that, when treated properly, are capable of healing themselves to a surprising degree. Still, a hundred years from now, all of us will have died. In the end, the only thing that will matter at all is our individual relationship with Jesus Christ, Son of God, Savior.

"My future is in God's hands," Justin said. "My children and their spouses-to-be, my future grandchildren—all in God's hands. I'm a good provider, a good parent-guide for them, but God is infinitely better. And He promises something I can never promise—He will never ever leave them."

Part of Justin's process of releasing his grip on his family was to host an extended family reunion. "I wanted us to rejoice together as a family—aunts, uncles, cousins, babies, everyone." Then he added, "There's nothing like cancer to get everyone to give top priority to getting together!"

Not everyone made it to the reunion, but that was all right too. Justin has also learned he doesn't have to control everything!

What changes have taken place in your life because of your cancer? What lessons have you learned? In what areas are you now able to make a difference?

"I no longer sleep late," Robert says. "I'm still young, but in lots of ways I feel much older than others my age. I push life aggressively. I don't put off until tomorrow what I can do today. I have every intention of living wisely and well."

An Eternal Perspective

So here you are, knowing what you know. Where do you go from here? How do you start living a refocused life?

Here's a great beginning point: bring praise to God by sharing the joy of your survival. Determine not to let a beautiful sunset go by unnoticed. Appreciate a garden running over with zucchini, a tree covered in brightly colored leaves even if they have to be raked up tomorrow, a baby's smile—or even tears. You have a special reason to drink in the bounty of life and to praise God for it.

And don't stop there. Determine that

- Whatever you do, you'll do it joyfully.
- Whenever and wherever possible, you'll relieve the suffering around you.
- You'll reach out and support anyone who is stumbling.
- You'll enjoy every single day God gives you and live it to its fullest.
- You'll love your family, your neighbor, your brothers and sisters in Christ. And most of all, you'll love your Heavenly Father.
- You'll celebrate any and every way you can. Sing.

Speak. Read Psalms. Maybe even write a few of your own.

- You'll create special moments—for yourself, yes, but also for those close to you.
- This day you'll enjoy the present. In the words of the psalmist, "This is the day the LORD has made; let us rejoice and be glad in it" (118:24).

"Here's one more to add to your list," Jen told me. "Don't ever, ever complain about getting older! I just celebrated my 38th birthday, and I was so happy that I could chalk up one more year. I can't wait until I'm an old lady and can say to my grandchildren, "Forty years ago, when I was diagnosed with cancer . . ."

"My wife and I walk our dogs in the park each afternoon," said Theo, "just for the sheer joy of being outside. We watch the clouds, admire the changing of the seasons in the trees, greet everyone we see, and say hello to their dogs. When we get home I give my wife a hug and say, 'Just imagine, Honey—I can still breathe!' And together we say a prayer of thanksgiving."

A refocused life is the life of a true survivor.

"I would not have chosen cancer, of course," Marlene says, "but I'll have to say that my experience with it truly changed my life for the better. I value family and friendships and the family of God in a whole new way. I have a peace I never knew before. I look back with gratitude to God for the wonderful life He has granted me, and I thank Him daily for allowing me the honor and joy of being salt and light in a unique way. There truly is life after cancer."

14

MORE THAN CONQUERORS

This morning I switched on the television set to watch the annual broadcast of the New Year's Day Rose Parade from Pasadena, California. Once, more years ago than I care to remember, my brand-new husband and I sat up all night on a sidewalk in Pasadena so we could have front-row seats from which to watch the Rose Parade pass by in all its real-life splendor. We could actually see the individual flowers that bedecked the floats that passed by just feet in front of us. Also discernable was the sweat on each band member's brow, the overdone makeup on the face of each grinning baton twirler, the intricate silver decorations on each horse's saddle. But watching it on television was so different. I couldn't make out any of those details. Instead, the camera panned back to display the entire parade as it snaked up Colorado Boulevard. The symmetry was perfect, the timing superb. What I had seen in person as real-life disconnected spots I now saw as a completed, unified, perfected whole. Not a misstep. Not a missed beat. Not a single wilted petal.

This is an imperfect analogy to be sure, but isn't it a little bit the way our lives must be seen through God's eyes? He is timeless. He sees the whole picture at once with all the pieces in place and running smoothly as a whole. And so His perspective is so much broader, so much more all-encompassing, so much more complete.

In Ps. 90:2 Moses wrote, "Before the mountains were born or you brought forth the earth and the world, from everlasting to everlasting you are God."

The fact that God exists "from everlasting to everlasting" is not only a profound theological statement but also a comforting and reassuring truth. He sees the whole picture of our lives and is with us through it all. Permeating every experience of every day is the sustaining grace of our loving, sovereign God.

In his great book *My Utmost for His Highest*, Oswald Chambers wrote, "When once you are rightly related to God by salvation and sanctification, remember that wherever you are, you are put there by God; and by the reaction of your life on the circumstances around you, you will fulfill God's purpose, as long as you keep in the light as God is in the light."[1]

In coming to the end of ourselves, we finally come to the beginning of our true and deepest selves. Only here can we find the One whose love gives substance and purpose to our lives.

That's not to say we've arrived. I would never say that about myself, and I doubt you would claim it for yourself either. No, we're constantly moving forward, growing, and maturing. New circumstances require new adjustments and more struggles and result in more growth. That's how it should be.

You may be healed supernaturally and miraculously. If so, praise God! On the other hand, God may simply have allowed you more time. Whether He grants you healing or not, He can and will give you His supernatural peace that passes all understanding. Yes, supernatural healing is wonderful. But supernatural peace is far, far greater.

"Each and every day is a gift from God," Nick says with conviction. "If I can point one person to God because of what I've gone through, then I'll know my life has not been in vain."

GREAT RICHES

Through your suffering, though grievous, you have amassed some great treasures. Just look at all that's piled into your treasure chest!

- Greater awareness of the sustaining power of God. "Praise be to the Lord, to God our Savior, who daily bears our burdens" (Ps. 68:19).
- Manifestations of Christ's work for all to see. "We have this treasure in jars of clay to show that this all-surpassing power is from God and not from us. We are hard pressed on every side, but not crushed; perplexed, but not in despair; persecuted, but not abandoned; struck down, but not destroyed" (2 Cor. 4:7-9).
- Understanding of your dependence on God. "'My grace is sufficient for you, for my power is made perfect in weakness.' Therefore I will boast all the more gladly about my weaknesses, so that Christ's power may rest on me" (2 Cor. 12:9).
- Character. "We also rejoice in our sufferings, because we know that suffering produces perseverance; perseverance, character; and character, hope" (Rom. 5:3-4).
- Understanding that the greatest good of the Christian life is not absence of pain but Christlikeness. "We always carry around in our body the death of Jesus, so that the life of Jesus may also be revealed in our body" (2 Cor. 4:10).
- Obedience and self-control.

Consider it pure joy, my brothers, whenever you face trials of many kinds, because you know that the testing of your faith develops perseverance. Perseverance must finish its work so that you may be mature and complete, not lacking anything. If any of you lacks wisdom, he should ask God, who gives generously to all without finding fault, and it will be given to him. But when he asks, he must believe and not doubt, because he who doubts is like a wave of the sea, blown and tossed by the wind. That man should not think he will receive anything from the Lord; he is a double-minded man, unstable in all he does *(James 1:2-8)*.

- The broken and contrite spirit God desires. "You do not delight in sacrifice, or I would bring it; you do not take pleasure in burnt offerings. The sacrifices of God are a broken spirit; a broken and contrite heart, O God, you will not despise" (Ps. 51:16-17).
- Minds focused on the grace to be revealed when we see Jesus Christ. "In this you greatly rejoice, though now for a little while you may have had to suffer grief in all kinds of trials. . . . Therefore, prepare your minds for action; be self-controlled; set your hope fully on the grace to be given you when Jesus Christ is revealed" (1 Pet. 1:6, 13).
- Strength and ability to comfort others.

Praise be to the God and Father of our Lord Jesus Christ, the Father of compassion and the God of all comfort, who comforts us in all our troubles, so that we can comfort those in any trouble with the comfort we ourselves have received from God. For just as the sufferings of Christ flow over into our lives, so also through Christ our comfort overflows. If we are distressed, it is for your comfort and salvation; if we are comforted, it is for your comfort, which produces in you patient endurance of the same sufferings we suffer. And our hope for you is firm, because we know that just as you share in our sufferings, so also you share in our comfort. We do not want you to be uninformed, brothers, about the hardships we suffered in the province of Asia. We were under great pressure, far beyond our ability to endure, so that we despaired even of life. Indeed, in our hearts we felt the sentence of death. But this happened that we might not rely on ourselves but on God, who raises the dead. He has delivered us from such a deadly peril, and he will deliver us. On him we have set our hope that he will continue to deliver us, as you help us by your prayers. Then many will give thanks on our behalf for the gracious favor granted us in answer to the prayers of many *(2 Cor. 1:3-11)*.

- Increased faith. "'I know the plans I have for you,' declares the LORD, 'plans to prosper you and not to harm you, plans to give you hope and a future'" (Jer. 29:11).
- An understanding of God's Care. "Record my lament; list my tears on your scroll—are they not in your record?" (Ps. 56:8).
- Stretched hope. "Though he slay me, yet will I hope in him; I will surely defend my ways to his face" (Job 13:15).

WE WIN!

Regardless of how we feel at any given time, we truly are the winners. Rom. 8:37-39 assures us that absolutely nothing can separate us from the love of God, which is in Christ Jesus our Lord. Because of Christ, we are not only survivors—we are more than conquerors.

The Bible's spotlight is on the end result. When it talks about suffering, it deals with it in the context of how God uses it in our lives.

Suffering forces us to the utter end of ourselves. And in its turn it allows us to begin a vital, fresh relationship with God. Having to face our own weaknesses, we realize just how much we take for granted.

A young teenager we'll call Luke was 13 when he was diagnosed with an aggressive form of leukemia. He and Myra's son were in the same class in school. Luke was already through treatment and was starting high school when Myra's cancer was diagnosed. Terrified at the thought of facing chemotherapy and radiation, and with everyone's horror stories ringing in her ears, Myra called Luke's mother. Luke and his mother bought Myra a copy of Philip Keller's book *A Shepherd Looks at the 23rd Psalm*. Myra read the book through that day and loved it.

A few days later, in the middle of the afternoon, the telephone rang. It was Luke. "I'm just calling to tell you that you're going to make it," the boy told Myra. "Don't be afraid of the chemotherapy or the radiation. It's no fun, and you're not going to like it, but look straight into the eyes of the nurse and the doctor, and know that you'll see Jesus in every person helping you. I know. I've been there." His words were like a word from the shepherd. Myra's fear melted.

Two years later Luke lost his battle with cancer and died.

Myra, however, was pronounced cured after three years. There's no evidence of any cancer in her body. Yet because of her bout with cancer, she continues to touch the lives of many people. One day in a Bible study, a woman tearfully asked for prayer for her 19-year-old nephew who had just been diagnosed with testicular cancer. "I'll pray for him!" Myra said. "And do you think it would be all right if I write to him? I have something I'd like to send him."

What Myra sent was the book Luke had sent her. And with it she included words of faith and encouragement, just as Luke had done for her.

Where is that young man today? And what's the condition of his soul? Myra doesn't know. But she does know where Luke is. His hope was in Christ, and he never missed an opportunity to say so. His faith strengthened and upheld Myra during her darkest days. And the day will come when Myra and Luke will rejoice together at the feet of Jesus. It's her prayer that the other young man will be there too.

God works according to His master plan. And it *will* be accomplished for His glory and our eternal good. And the time will come when we'll all shout in unison, *Thank You, Lord!*

HOME AT LAST

The world offers us passing pleasures (Heb. 11:25) that are dependent upon our circumstances. Those pleasures can feel quite good, to be sure—but they don't last. That's because circumstances change. The Lord Jesus offers us something quite different—full and lasting joy (John 15:11). Joy is inward and, unlike passing pleasures, is not disturbed by environment. While pleasure is always changing, joy is constant. Worldly delights are often followed by depression. Not so with true joy, for it's grounded in Jesus Christ, who "is the same yesterday and today and forever" (Heb. 13:8).

In his letter to the church at Philippi the apostle Paul wrote, "To me, to live is Christ and to die is gain" (1:21).

Paul was a survivor. He survived death threats, shipwrecks, poisonous snakes, mobs, prison, beatings, some unknown physical affliction, illness, stoning—you name it; he survived it. He wanted to live, of course. Yet he had no illusions about where his home really was.

Hold this world lightly, for it's not your home. When you arrive in heaven, one thing will be immediately and wonderfully obvious: *Heaven is what you were made for! You're home at last!* Allow yourself the great freedom of thinking of and rejoicing over that joyous homecoming.

Until then, grow and blossom, then plentifully produce the fruits of the Spirit: "The fruit of the Spirit is love, joy, peace, patience, kindness, goodness, faithfulness, gentleness and self-control. Against such things there is no law" (Gal. 5:22-23).

You are a survivor!
Congratulations!
Live well!

Appendix

Helpful Resources

The World Wide Web is a wonderful boon to those of us who want to have up-to-date information at our fingertips. The resources and addresses that follow are intended to help you gain access to such information. But with that access comes a warning: An awful lot of what is available on the Web is at best unreliable and at worst a con game preying on the sick and vulnerable. So be very careful when you go on-line. Make sure the site is from a reputable source, keeping in mind that names can sometimes be deceiving. Be particularly careful about giving out sensitive and personal information and especially your credit card number.

That said, here are some highly reputable and extremely helpful sources to begin with:

- Association of Cancer Online Resources
  www.medinfo.org
  This site provides direct links to the archives of cancer support groups such as BMT-Talk and Hem-Onc. It also provides links to CancerNet. (See listing for CancerNet.)
- American Cancer Society
  www.cancer.org
  1599 Clifton Road N.E.
  Atlanta, GA 30329
  800-ACS-2345
  Both by telephone and web site, the American Cancer Society has a great deal to offer. The web site, for instance, has links to such topics as promising cancer treatments and cancer wellness books. It also has a

131

feature that allows you to ask questions on many topics, including diagnosis, treatment, and the availabili-
ty of information and materials.

- The Best Doctors in America
  www.bestdoctors.com
  E-mail: info@bestdoctors.com
  Phone: 888-DOCTORS
  Fax: 803-648-7240
  This resource directory is grouped by regions and, at
  $95 per volume, is quite pricey. In addition, it charges
  a fee for a personalized search for doctors specializing
  in a particular area. However, the book is available in
  some public libraries and may well be worth a look.
- CancerNet
  cancernet.nci.nih.gov
  This includes the up-to-date research and treatment
  summaries on various forms of cancer from the National Cancer Institute. (See the following listing.)
- National Cancer Institute
  www.cancer.gov
  800-4-CANCER
  Through its telephone service, the National Cancer
  Institute offers a wide range of information, including
  links to such topics as research and ongoing drug and
  treatment trials. Its web site is informative and easy to
  use. It offers a number of free publications about cancer and its treatments.
- The National Library of Medicine
  www.nim.nih.gov
  888-346-3656
  301-594-5983
  8699 Rockville Pike
  Bethesda, MD 20894
  Publication: MEDLINE. This can be retrieved from
  the World Wide Web at the following address:
  www.ncbi.nlm.nih.gov/PubMed
  This is a web retrieval system developed by the Na-

tional Library of Medicine that provides free access to MEDLINE, a huge database of journal articles that can be searched according to specific diseases or types of cancer. It has various features that help you search for what you want and need.

NOTES

Introduction
1. C. S. Lewis, *A Grief Observed* (London: Farber and Farber, 1961), 25.

Chapter 2
1. Eric Sabo, "Hit the Health Jackpot," *McCall's*, March 2001, 90.
2. Jeremy Geffen, *The Journey Through Cancer* (New York: Crown Publishing, 2000), 41.

Chapter 4
1. Jill Carroll, "Regulators Crack Down of Web's New Miracle Cure: Colloidal Silver," *Wall Street Journal*, June 14, 2001, B1.
2. David Sneed and Sharon Sneed, *The Hidden Agenda: A Critical View of Alternative Medical Therapies* (Nashville: Thomas Nelson Publishers, 1991), 62-77.
3. Larry Burkett, *Hope When It Hurts: A Personal Testimony of How to Deal with the Impact of Cancer* (Chicago: Moody Press, 1998), 82.
4. Jack Canfield et al., *Chicken Soup for the Surviving Soul: 101 Healing Stories of Courage and Inspiration* (Deerfield Beach, Fla.: Health Communications, 1996).

Chapter 5
1. Jason Winters, *Killing Cancer* (Las Vegas, Nev.: Vinton Publishing, 1980), n.p.
2. Look for these and other helpful contacts in the resource list found in the Appendix.
3. Larry Burkett, *Hope When It Hurts*, 159-61.

Chapter 7
1. 1994 National Cancer Institute Workshop on Cancer Pain, as reported in "Management of Cancer Pain," a publication of the United States Department of Health and Human Services.

Chapter 9
1. C. S. Lewis, *A Grief Observed*, 5.
2. Philip Yancey, *Where Is God When It Hurts?* (Grand Rapids: Zondervan Publishing House, 1990), 99.
3. Ibid., 230.

4. Lewis, *The Problem of Pain,* 39-42.

Chapter 14

1. Oswald Chambers, *My Utmost for His Highest* (New York: Dodd, Mead and Company, 1935), 231.